Advance Praise for *What Kind of Mother*

"*What Kind of Mother* is a poignant, brilliantly-written evocation of what it means to come to terms with a child's addiction and mental illness, and in the process one's own struggles and history overcoming secrecy and shame, and how they conspire to destroy families from within. Absolutely unforgettable—this is a story that will stay with me forever."
—Elissa Altman, author of *Permission: The New Memoirist and the Courage to Create* and *Motherland: A Memoir of Love, Loathing, and Longing*

"Incredibly warm and funny and tender, this is a riveting story about what happens when we have to face our worst fears—about ourselves and the children we love. With wry humor and a wildly compelling voice, *What Kind of Mother* dares to do the taboo: to talk about what happens when things don't go at all according to the plan. It's a book about taking the blinders off and a very moving love story. I could not put it down."
—Susan Conley, author of *Landslide* and *The Foremost Good Fortune: A Memoir*

"Sandler's memoir delves into the poignant realization of a mother's limitations in shielding her family from life's hardships, offering a raw and honest exploration of love, mental illness, and the struggle for redemption. What she believed she could not control she can and has controlled this narrative in a direction of pure heart. *What Kind of Mother* is a gem . . . this is art, this is literature with a capital L, literature built on the foundation of emotion, the very thing that allows any reader to connect to."

—Morgan Talty, author of *Night of the Living Rez: Stories* and *Fire Exit: A Novel*

"*What Kind of Mother* is a heartbreakingly vulnerable and sobering portrayal of what it is like to watch your child spiral into addiction and reckon with the life-altering effects of mental illness. With searing honesty, Judy Sandler takes us into her complex journey of retracing the family history and parenting decisions that might make her culpable in the ongoing story of her son's struggle to find equilibrium."

—Melanie Brooks, author of *A Hard Silence: One Daughter Remaps Family, Grief, and Faith when HIV/AIDS Changes It All*

"The narrative becomes a source of solace, forging connections among those who share in the silent struggles of nurturing and supporting adult children with mental health challenges."

—David Goodman, MD, Johns Hopkins University School of Medicine

WHAT KIND OF MOTHER

CONNECTIVE TISSUE

A Health Humanities and Narrative Medicine Series
Renée K. Nicholson, Series Editor

CONNECTIVE TISSUE is a series in health humanities and narrative medicine that illuminates lived experiences with health, illness, and medicine. This series explores innovative approaches to healthcare by integrating expressive arts and humanities practices into therapeutic settings and generating works of creative writing that artfully render stories of illness, disability, and the journey to well-being.

Dizzy: A Memoir
Rachel Weaver

What Kind of Mother: A Reckoning
Judy Sandler

WHAT KIND *of* MOTHER

A Reckoning

Judy Sandler

West Virginia University Press | Morgantown

First edition published 2026 by West Virginia University Press
Printed in the United States of America
ISBN 978-1-959000-80-8 (paperback) ISBN 978-1-959000-81-5 (epub)
ISBN 978-1-959000-82-2 (PDF)

Library of Congress Control Number: 2026013700

Cover design by Zoe Norvell
Book design by Kelley Galbreath
Cover images by Serge Filimonov / Stocksy and Jesse Weinberg / Stocksy

For EU safety/GPSR concerns, please direct inquiries to WVUPress@mail.wvu.edu or our physical mailing address at West Virginia University Press / PO Box 6295 / West Virginia University / Morgantown

FOR SKIP

and for Alex, Lucy, and Noah

They say addiction might be linked to bipolar disorder.
It's the chemicals in our brains, they say. I got the
wrong chemicals, Ma. Or rather, I don't get enough
of one or the other. They have a pill for it. They have
an industry. They make millions. Did you know
people get rich off of sadness?

I want to meet the millionaire of American sadness.
I want to look him in the eye, shake his hand, and say,
"It's been an honor to serve my country."

—Ocean Vuong
On Earth We're Briefly Gorgeous

AUTHOR'S NOTE

The people and places in this book are real. In order to protect their privacy, some names in the book and most places have been changed.

The names of the following locations in the book are pseudonyms: Alliance House, Compass Rose, Nature Quest Wilderness Therapy, Oceanside Psychiatric Hospital, St. Mark's Hospital, and Thorne Street. All other places and locations remain unchanged. Passages from James's journals, with his permission, and the author's journal, emails, and texts have been printed as they originally appeared.

PREFACE

Every family has a defining narrative, a story you learn not by the telling but rather through a mysterious alchemy of watching and osmosis. You learn it more from what was *not* said than by what was spoken directly to you. Maybe you learn by watching your siblings, witnessing what got them into trouble and what provoked from your father, at the dinner table, "Hey, did you hear what your brother did at school today?" What does your mother repeat to your father, and what does she keep a secret? By the time I was ten years old, I knew the family myth: We were a perfect family, consumed by what the neighbors and my father's colleagues at the newspaper thought of us, ever mindful of the expectations for a family "like us." If we had difficulties in math class in school, felt left out by our social life, or had the burning desire to break out of the mold, we learned to conceal our feelings. Things like that did not happen to families like ours. No psychiatric hospitals or psychologists for any of us.

My sister loved cats, but no one else in the family did. My parents answered a cat-for-sale ad in the newspaper and drove to Pennsylvania from our home in Maryland to find my sister a white Persian. A few years later, I was a wiry kid in a T-shirt and shorts, running up the two steps in front of our house, and there was Trouble, tucked between our stone steps, lying motionless. At first, I didn't think anything of it. Cats sleep on the steps all the time. But Trouble didn't look like she was breathing. I nudged her with my tennis shoe. Nothing. And here is a symptom of the family secret: instead of running inside and begging my mother to get Trouble to the vet, I continued on my way down the stone path, through the front door, and never told my mother or sister that Trouble was dead. Why did I do this? Because our family's legend meant everything was alright in our home. I would not be the one to break the code. Deaths happened in other families, illness too. To the outside world, which was apparently always judging us, we were the kind of family pictured on the front of a Life cereal box. The secret of a dead cat is a small omission in some mythologies, but decades later, the power of that secret would grow. This time, I wasn't a daughter or a little sister; I was a mother, and my son kept tripping and falling off the path of success my parents had paved for me, and that I had paved for him. And for years, I pretended it wasn't happening.

My father was a professional writer, and an excellent one. He passed on to me an impossible, two-sided trait: an allegiance to keep the family code, but also the inherent need to write. In her book, *Permission: The New Memoirist and the Courage to Create*, Elissa Altman writes, "No other emotion prompts secrecy like shame." I was ashamed that I found the dead cat. I was ashamed my son suffered from mental illness and addiction. And I was ashamed that I was ashamed. What I needed to do was face the truth and accept it. For a good while, I believed that if I learned everything I could about addiction and mental health, I could solve his problems; I could fix him. As I began to write this book, I came to understand that it wasn't my son who needed to be fixed; it was me. I needed to surrender and accept him for who he was.

The most difficult part of writing this book was not the remembering or the making of sentences. It was granting myself permission to tell the story, to put into the world something about my family that didn't look like the picture on the cereal box. It took me many, many years to be able to say to my son, "I don't think I need your permission to write this story because it's my story. But I would like your blessing." Only recently did my son tell me, "I trust you to tell your story and not mine."

I have done my best not to tell my son's story because that is his to share with you one day, and I hope he does. Memory does not play back like a script or a tape recorder. Rather, it is more like a tide, leaving certain images behind, washing others away. What remains are the stories I've picked up and held, like shells, along the way. The people in these pages are real, but with few exceptions, their names have been changed to protect their privacy. Likewise, the names of certain places and organizations have also been changed. The dates are accurate, according to journals I kept, emails, texts, and other clues as to when the events occurred. Excerpts from James's journals have been reprinted with his permission. The structure of the chapters titled "I'm Glad You Asked" was influenced by Maggie Smith's book *You Could Make This Place Beautiful*. Her work reminded me that when I ask and answer my own questions, I can be both vulnerable and truthful on the page.

I offer this story as an example of what can happen when shame is converted into understanding and communication, when the illusion of control is let go, and when knowledge becomes a kind of power I am able to put into words. I hope the book gives others the courage to shout their stories from the rooftops.

WHAT KIND OF MOTHER

I CONFESS

I didn't recognize my own son in the parking lot of the Adult Crisis Stabilization Unit. His jaunty trot now a shuffling gait. A thin cap, knotted at the top, pulled over his head. I wanted to ask this man, "Have you seen my son? Do you know where my devilish boy went? Excuse me, you seem a lot like him. Yet, you can't possibly be him." We don't intentionally wound our children with such questions. So, I said, "I like your hat." And he said, "Thanks, the night nurse made it for me. Out of a glove."

KINDLING

NATURE QUEST WILDERNESS THERAPY (JAMES'S JOURNAL)

SOMEWHERE IN SOUTHERN UTAH, JANUARY 9, 2012

Having a large and close friend group (not complaining or bragging) has been hard in terms of deciding who is an intimate friend and who are the people I pass by and say hi to occasionally. I first drank with my French exchange friend when I was 13. I started using ecstasy when I was 16. I started using LSD when I was 16 also. I experimented with opium and DMT when I was 17. When I went to college at 19, I tried cocaine and ketamine, and nitrous. I've been constantly smoking nearly every day since I was a sophomore in high school.

DIRECTIONS FOR HOW TO PLAY

This is what I learned from my father: There is one way to be in this world, and it's not complicated. Go to school, do exceptionally well at whatever cost, attend an Ivy League college, preferably the University of Pennsylvania, choose a career that will enable you to support yourself financially, marry someone Jewish of the opposite gender, have children, repeat the cycle, generation after generation.

He taught me the emotions of anger, sadness, and frustration are to be experienced quickly and numbed away. My father showed me how to ignore conflict, be it sibling rivalry, separation anxiety, or the emergence of obsessive-compulsive disorder in my older sister. I gathered we did not discuss these things in public. We barely talked about them in the private confines of our home.

My father was a big deal. You couldn't go out to lunch with him in Baltimore without someone stopping at the table and asking, "Are you Gilbert Sandler?" He shook hands with everyone and kissed favorite waitresses at the Center Club. Every Jewish person in Baltimore knew my father, and if they didn't know him, they knew someone who knew him. Or they had read something that he wrote. Or they had found an error in his last column in the *Baltimore Sun*. Or they wanted to know why he didn't include their family in his last book, *Jewish Baltimore*. Or they knew some fact he didn't include in *Small Town Baltimore*, his book about the city during the Depression

"How did you miss that, Gilbert?" a woman once asked him while she stood behind our lunch table, grilling him about his recent piece on the beginnings of the well-known department stores in Baltimore. "Ach," he told me after she left, "she's crazy."

In the board game called Life, according to my father, I started at "Go" and went around and around the board, abiding by his rules. He told me that quitting is never an option. He told me where to go to college, what my major should be, and what I wanted to be when I grew up. It was only recently that I realized there were other ways to play this game. My slow learning has been at the expense of my own children. At the expense, most of all, of my oldest son, James.

I am aware now there are many different ways to make the trip around the board. But in raising James, I often reverted to the rules my father taught me. James picked up on these lessons, the not-so-subtle messages about what success should look like. Something in James, a predisposition in his DNA perhaps, has always rejected the speed at which I suggest he move, the endgame I was steering him toward. And so, in the same way clear vinegar poured into a child's model of a volcano packed with baking powder is destined to erupt, James began to bubble over.

THE CABALLEROS ARE COMING

DECEMBER 1972

I am ten, too old to be put to bed by my father, but I climb into my bed and wait for him to come upstairs to put me to bed anyway. I have a chin-up bar at the top of my door because I am into strength conditioning at ten years old. I hear his footsteps on the wooden stairwell. I know the difference between the sound of his footsteps and the sound of Mom's footsteps. Then he pauses at the end of the hallway. I wait. He takes a running start and picks up speed as he approaches my bedroom door, the last one at the end of the hallway on the right. He jumps up to my chin-up bar, grabs hold of it, and swings his body onto my bed. He lands next to me. "Shhh," he tells me. "Shhh, we have to be quiet. The caballeros are coming. We have to hide."

He puts the pillow over both of our heads and makes clicking sounds with his mouth that sound like hoofbeats trotting by. Then he says, "You seen 'em? A man and a kid. We're coming back for 'em." More trotting sounds until the horse runs off in the distance.

We are safe. He removes the pillow from on top of our faces.

"Gilbert!" my mom calls from their bedroom across the hall. "Stop that! She's too old for that!"

Never too old for that.

SHAME ON ME

MARCH 1976

As soon as Dr. Adams walked out of my ninth grade English classroom, probably to have another smoke, everyone in the class began to share answers on the pop quiz on *Macbeth*. I sat between my best friend, Emily, and a boy who had been in my class since third grade, Taylor. Each of us had an English quiz on our desks—ten multiple-choice questions. Everyone knew Dr. Adams's class was a joke. We were in ninth grade at an independent school in Baltimore, and he could have been a college professor. No one had any idea what he was talking about when he lectured.

"What do you have for number three?" I didn't even whisper the question. Others around me were trading the actual quizzes back and forth. Just as Emily leaned over to compare her number three with mine, Dr. Adams stormed back into the room.

We got quiet but not quickly enough. In the odd, jerky way he moved his body, his head wound up facing me, and his eyes landed on my quiz. The entire class had shared answers, but Dr. Adams's wild blue eyes focused only on me.

"Who are you talking to?" he snapped.

"No one," I lied badly, staring right at him. But it was too late. Emily had already changed her answer on the quiz to match my number three, and it turned out to be the wrong answer.

Dr. Adams took a few long steps toward Emily and Taylor. He snatched up their quizzes, then swiped mine from my desk, and placed them in his leather briefcase. "After class," he leaned in, his breath warm and smelling of cigarettes, "go directly to your advisors. They will handle it from here."

"But . . ." Taylor attempted to explain the obvious, that everyone in the class was cheating. But it was no use.

Mr. McKnight, my ninth-grade advisor, suggested I confess to my parents as soon as I got home because he told me, "I will be calling them this evening. And I think it would be best if they heard it from you first."

I could explain the situation to my mother, and she was likely to let it go. But not my dad. Cheating was cheating, and teachers were teachers. There was not an in-between with him. I was going to have to tell him what happened without any excuses about how strange Dr. Adams was, what a joke the class was, or how everyone was doing it but I got caught.

My father predictably walked into the house at 6:00 in the evening, headed for his study on the first floor of our contemporary brick house in Baltimore, wrote, watched *World News Tonight*, and read that day's edition of the *Baltimore Sun*, the paper he wrote for, until dinner. My mother cooked flank steak (main course), rice (always a starch), and spinach (a healthy vegetable) in the kitchen, which was right next to his study. They called back and forth to one another about their day without being in the same room together, somehow communicating through the walls.

My father's study was a warm, intimate, bookcase-lined room that smelled like a dry cork. He was a collector of things—nothing was too insignificant—and above his desk, a wooden shelf ran the length of one side of the room, where sat my cast from fifth grade when I broke my arm at summer camp, his green combat helmet from World War II, his University of Pennsylvania diploma, many letters of alumni recognition for his work raising money and acting as an alumni recruiter for the school, and a collection of small, red and silver tin containers that used to hold typewriter ribbons. I spied new, arcane objects every time I looked at the shelf. But that's not why I was standing at the door this time.

My father wore a white button-down shirt, khaki pants, and a bow tie every day. He was already seated in his glossy, black Penn alumni chair in front of his electric typewriter. "Hi, Dad," I said, trying to determine his mood.

"Hey, Jude!"

Pretty chipper.

"How's school today?" he asked.

"Well, actually, that's what I'm here to talk about. Not so good. Mr. McKnight is going to call you later. So I want to talk to you before he calls."

My father peered over his thick, black-rimmed glasses. His fingers stopped tapping at the keys. "Mr. McKnight, your advisor?" He stood up from his chair and looked straight at me. But he never moved from behind his typewriter.

"Yeah, Dad. It's so dumb. It was like, we were in English with Dr. Adams, and he left the room in the middle of a quiz. No teacher leaves in the middle of a quiz. But Dr. Adams is so dumb."

"Don't call your teachers dumb. They're not dumb. They are your teachers, that's why they are there. To teach you." My father's voice was low, steady, and firm. He held his glasses in one hand and leaned against his desk with his other hand, staring down at me from behind his typewriter.

"Dad, Dr. Adams doesn't teach. I don't even know what he's saying. Anyway, what Mr. McKnight is going to tell you is that Emily and I were talking about the answer to a question on this stupid quiz when Dr. Adams was out of the room, and then he came back in, and like, everyone in the class was talking and sharing answers, but he caught Emily and me, and now we're the only ones in the class getting in trouble. It's so not fair, Dad. Don't you get it?" Warm tears welled up in my eyes, and my throat tightened. I couldn't talk to him anymore, but I dared not leave the doorway.

My father didn't yell at me. He didn't even move. He stared straight at me when I met his brown eyes, tears now dripping down my cheeks. I wish he had let loose on me or told me to go to my room, shouting after me about how disappointed he was and how he knew I could do better. I wish he could have called my mother from the kitchen into the study and grilled me with questions about the class and Dr. Adams and what the hell was going on in that class anyway. I wish I could have sobbed and told him how ashamed I was, how I couldn't live up to his ridiculously high expectations, and that all of his children couldn't be shining pillars of the community all the time. We couldn't be perfect examples of what children should look like and be and do. I wish I had screamed at him, "People make mistakes!"

But nothing like that happened.

Silence filled his study.

He stared down at me, frozen in his stance behind the typewriter. “Look at me,” my father said, even though I was already staring at him. “I never want to hear about this again. You will never do this again. You will never cheat again. Do you understand?”

I nodded slowly, sniffling.

“Answer me.”

“I understand,” I whispered with hot, wet breath.

He adjusted his glasses on his face, glanced back at his typewriter, and threaded a piece of white paper through the guide.

“You can go now,” he said softly to his typewriter.

“I’m sorry, Dad.” I turned and walked out of his study, through the den, and upstairs to my bedroom. If my mother overheard the conversation from the kitchen, she never let on, and we did not discuss it later at dinner, or ever.

One more thing. Mr. McKnight never called my parents.

NATURE QUEST WILDERNESS THERAPY

SOMEWHERE IN SOUTHERN UTAH, JANUARY 9, 2012

I was born in Baltimore, Maryland on November 25th, 1991. (Thanksgiving.) I have lived in Baltimore County until I graduated high school and attended Colorado College for Freshman year. I have attended Friends School of Baltimore from kindergarten to senior year. I've worked as a busboy at a restaurant, a soccer camp counselor, and a landscaper over the past three summers. I want to complete college and possibly graduate school in hopes of living a happy, independent life. I've been talking to a therapist since freshman year of high school to deal with family issues involving pot use and substance use in general.

KEEP MOVING

MARCH 1969

I grew up in the sixties and seventies in Mt. Washington, an old, tree-lined, white, upper-middle-class neighborhood in Baltimore City, where we played touch football in the street. The cracks in the black asphalt and two streetlights on either side of the street marked the goalposts. When someone yelled, "Car!" we ambled toward the curb. In the evenings after dinner, those same kids opened their front doors, flashlights in hand, for Kick the Can, which lasted well past dark. On the rare occasion that I was bored, I called my friend Emily, who lived one house away from mine, and we agreed to meet in front of Ronnie's driveway, the one in between our houses, where we sat on the curb, digging dirt with a stick out of the crack in the sidewalk, and said, "What do you wanna do?"

Inside my house, my father clacked away at the electric typewriter in his study. He had a small black-and-white television in there, a nine-inch portable thing, and I wanted nothing more than to sit on the black leather sofa with him and watch the fuzzy screen, but my father's rule was no television on weekdays. No one challenged this rule; no one even raised their voice in my childhood home. As far as I can remember, there was little reason to shout, as it appeared to me that there were no conflicts in my house.

I remember only one time when my father lost his temper. We were having dinner in our light-filled dining room, which had a brick floor and white walls, a hutch along one of them. My older sister made the mistake of talking back to my mother after my mother had questioned whether it was a good idea for her to have seconds on the flank steak.

"Go to your room," my father told her calmly from the head of the table, then poked a bite of steak with his fork. He was looking at his food; all we could see were thinning strands of dark hair on his otherwise balding head.

"No," my sister said, "I'm not finished eating dinner." She stared directly at my father, her wavy, shoulder-length hair framing her face, her white, uniform button-down shirt open at the collar, her green plaid skirt unbuttoned at the waist, spread across her chair.

I thought maybe I hadn't heard her correctly. My legs swung back and forth under the table while I held my breath and stared at her. I put my fork down on my plate and waited. I knew there was going to be trouble. I glanced at my brother next to me, but he was concentrating on shoveling food into his mouth, his arm moving robotically from his plate to his face.

My father held his fork in the air, pulled back his chair, which made a scraping sound on the brick, and took a few steps toward my sister. "I said, go to your room."

My sister look startled, then rose from her chair and took off running for her room, through the living room, up the short flight of wooden steps.

My father ran after her, still clenching the fork in his fist, although I do not believe he would have hurt her.

I heard the door to my sister's room slam shut, then my father returned to the table. He sat down at his place, put the cloth napkin back in his lap, glanced up at my mother, brother, and me, as if to ask, "What? Is something wrong?" and resumed eating his dinner. He wasn't sweating, his button-down shirt was still tucked into his khaki pants, and he wasn't even out of breath. He looked remarkably calm considering the sprint he had just completed.

No one spoke about my sister's back talk. My mother, father, brother, and I finished eating dinner in silence.

STAIN

My quiet, reliable home, where no one ever raised their voice and life predictably moved ahead day by day, left a fingerprint on my brain. Well, maybe more like a stain. My father's silent agreement with my mother, "No fighting in front of the children," created an illusion in our house; it was as though we lived under the spell of a magic trick.

Only after the magician said, "Abracadabra" and pulled the scarf away did I realize that my brother, sister, and I feared confrontation and still do not respond well to raised voices. Now, as a mother, I realize I tried to recreate my childhood home, one where I perpetuated my parents' myth that if my two boys, my daughter, my husband, and I looked clean and dressed appropriately, we were good people. If we read a lot and didn't watch television on weekdays, we were smart. If we didn't raise our voices in public, we were a close family. If we didn't discuss mental illness in the family, it didn't exist.

It seems an unconscious decision on my part to pass the myth of my childhood on to my children. In doing so, I did nothing to dilute the stain. If I want to drown myself in guilt now, I can wonder if my ambition for my children to excel at sports, to be academically excellent, and to become exceptional at something, anything, could have triggered James's substance use disorder and mental illness. I wonder if he reflects on his childhood and believes he was in some way traumatized by the pressure to become someone he did not want to be. My rational brain, and experts in the field of psychiatry, tell me that although childhood neglect, sexual and physical abuse, emotional abuse, and the death of a parent can trigger bipolar disorder, so can brain chemistry, genetics, and drug and alcohol abuse.

No matter how I turn the kaleidoscope of James's childhood, I would not use the word "abuse" to describe anything that happened to him under my watch. Do I have regrets as a mother? Of course. But I don't believe the ghosts of my father's expectations became the root of James's diagnosis.

I am working on changing the narrative in my head to the refrain, "It's no one's fault."

I am learning how to dissolve the stain from the fingerprint of my childhood.

BEST-LAID PLANS

NOVEMBER 1991

In my sixth month of pregnancy with James, my husband and I attended Lamaze classes for eight weeks in a large, airy room at the Jewish Community Center in Baltimore. With several other couples, we practiced methods of breathing, concentration, meditation, and relaxation. These techniques were supposed to ease the pain of childbirth when all hell broke loose in the delivery room. I remember watching a movie of a woman giving birth using these Lamaze methods. The woman was calm, never screamed or shouted, and never cursed at her partner or the doctors. She didn't even look like she was in pain; she appeared to be in a trance. I wanted to believe if my husband and I practiced our breathing enough times, this woman could be me when it came time to give birth.

But nothing like that happened. My water broke in the middle of brunch at a friend's house. I remember shoveling in forks of scrambled eggs, spreading cream cheese on an everything bagel, and suddenly feeling a warm gush of fluid between my legs. My underwear was soaked, as was the fabric-covered chair. "Oh my god, gross," is what I'm sure I whispered to myself. I searched the room for Daniel and spotted him standing near a window, sipping a mimosa from a tall glass, chatting with a dark-haired woman. "We have to go," I mouthed to him, after catching his eyes with mine.

Placing his glass on the windowsill, he walked directly to me, helped me out of the chair to which I believed I might be stuck, and, apologizing to our friends on our way out of their apartment, we hurried out the door. For the next ten hours, in an attempt to get my cervix to dilate enough to start an epidural, Daniel and I paced the white tile floors of the maternity halls of Baltimore's Sinai Hospital. "Breathe," my husband whispered quietly in my ear as another contraction gripped my body. "Just take a long slow breath."

"Fuck off!" I fumed at him between gritted teeth, and I meant it.

This was not going at all as I planned. Later, my father-in-law told me that from the comfort of the waiting room, he could hear me shout profanities and moan in pain straight through the walls. Finally, as I lay flat on my back on the hospital bed, an anesthesiologist told me the possible side effects of the epidural: "If we miss the spot in your back with the needle, you will have the worst headache of your life."

"Hurry," I told him between the contractions.

The epidural numbed the blinding pain of the contractions, but it also slowed them down. I was on my thirtieth hour of labor when James's heart rate dropped, as indicated by a terrifying beeping sound on a monitor to which I was attached by black wires. Within seconds, everything was a blur of motion, a rush of blue and green hospital gowns, doctors in shower caps. Orderlies sped me down a hallway on a gurney, my husband keeping up next to me, holding my hand.

When I heard him say, "I consent," I barely had time to wonder what part of my body or the baby's body he was consenting to. In a matter of minutes, I was in a small, cold room and could no longer feel anything from my waist down except for blessed relief. I was wide awake but numb.

My husband announced from behind his mask, "There's your intestine!" And then, "This is amazing!"

Within two minutes, my obstetrician pulled a baby from a four-inch-long, horizontal slit about three inches below my belly button.

I heard a wail, slow at first, like a cackle, then a loud, steady cry. It felt as though a lid finally turned; the jar was, at last, opened.

"He's okay?" I asked, staring up at a large fluorescent light.

"He's perfect," my husband said.

"He's great," my doctor confirmed before cutting the umbilical cord with surgical scissors. The nurses swaddled James in a cotton blanket and brought him back to me after I had been stitched up, attached to a morphine drip, and told, "Press this little button, sweetheart, when you feel pain."

CARD TRICKS

When Daniel and I talk about James's childhood, we try to figure out where we may have gone wrong. Years spread out before us like a face-down deck of cards, smoothly fanned out across a table. We pick a random card, turn it over, and wonder if it was the trigger. But we have never found the right card. It's never clear to us that one event in James's life caused him to later do the things he did. Daniel and I could turn over all the cards, one by one, examine the entire deck, and still never have an answer to the question, "Was this the card?"

Like my plan for James's birth, our life with him now is not the way I thought it would be. I can hold the things that went as planned with James in the palm of one hand, while everything else tumbles over like a house of cards.

HIDING

OCTOBER 1999

"I'm not wearing that pretty dress!" Julia shouted in her best loud voice. She was five years old, jumping up and down on her bed, wearing only her tiny underwear. Wiry and small, it was a wonder she didn't fly off the bed.

"I want to wear my purple velvet pants with the butterflies," she begged from midair.

I sighed deeply because what Julia wore that evening to my mother-in-law's Erev Yom Kippur dinner was the least of my worries.

"Fine, Julia," I said, careful to disguise the tension I felt about dinner that evening.

While I was upstairs getting James and Julia dressed in their holiday best, Daniel waited downstairs on the sofa in the family room, staring at the television. News anchors' voices filled the room with white noise. Already dressed in khaki pants, a pink button-down shirt, a paisley bow tie, and a navy jacket, Daniel looked handsome, clean, and put together. But I knew better. Recently diagnosed with bipolar type II disorder, my husband's red-rimmed eyes and hard-set jaw exposed the efforts he made to keep himself together. All evening, I would help him hide.

It was early October in Baltimore. Every year around the Jewish holidays, I expected the weather to have cooled off and the humidity to have lifted. But it never did. The tips of the leaves on the trees defied the high temperatures as if they had been dipped, kicking and screaming, into a square of gold paint in a paint box. After the fifteen-minute drive from our house in rural Stevenson to my mother-in-law's building in suburban Pikesville, we stood as a family of four in front of the hunter-green door.

"Let me do the knocker!" James begged, jumping up to reach the brass lion's head.

"No, James!" Julia shouted. "Let me do it. Daddy, pick me up so I can do the knocker!"

I glanced at Daniel. He closed his eyes, causing a few tears to leak down his cheeks. Even this was too much for him to deal with right now.

"Stop it." I was careful not to raise my voice.

Placing my hands under the armpits of James's navy blazer, I lifted him up to the brass knocker. He gave it a hard bang.

"You can do it next time, Julia." James glanced down at Julia with some empathy.

After I placed him back on his feet, he reached behind the back of his blazer and tucked in his shirt, which had come out of his khaki pants when I picked him up. His straight, chestnut-brown hair fell in a perfect bowl cut around his face. Julia folded her arms over her chest and stuck out her bottom lip. Daniel stood behind us like a shadow.

My mother-in-law opened the door. She was a young seventy-three-year-old woman, well dressed in black pants, a silk shirt, and a scarf arranged fashionably around her neck. She always wore an apron when she cooked, and tonight was no exception. James and Julia ran into her open arms, causing her to stumble backward. She laughed at their enthusiasm, "Well, welcome! Come in, kids!"

The house was warm and smelled like roasting meat. I felt Daniel behind me, robotically taking off his coat and hanging it in the hall closet. He was there but not there. Daniel's father, Joe, stood behind my mother-in-law, waiting for the commotion to end. He smiled his warm smile without opening his mouth and nodded slowly as if to say, "Here they come. I am a lucky man indeed."

After James and Julia wriggled out of their coats and tossed them over the back of a sofa, they ran down the hall to find their cousins. Daniel's Dad kissed the top of my head and wrapped his arms around his son. Out of everyone in this family, Joe was the one who seemed to sympathize with Daniel's depression the most. He'd drive to our house each morning and stay the entire day with Daniel in his home office, talking quietly with him, reassuring him that this storm was going to pass. Joe was the only one in the family, including me, who wasn't playing the hiding game.

He didn't care who knew, and he didn't care if Daniel needed to quit his job as a fund manager at T. Rowe Price. His only concern was his son's well-being, while the rest of us—Daniel's mother, his sister, his sister's husband, our own children, and me—wanted him to get better but didn't know how to help.

My mother-in-law moved some flowers around in a vase in the kitchen. Everything in the condo—the tan-and-red-patterned wallpaper in the family room, the down sofas slip-covered in chintz, the plates painted with delicate flowers hanging from the walls—should have felt comforting. On previous visits to this very room, all of it felt warm and welcoming. But at this moment, we were not fitting in. I was on high alert on the edge of the plush sofa, sitting between Daniel, his older sister, and her husband. It was like being at the state fair and losing at Whac-A-Mole.

At any moment, I knew Daniel could devolve into a wet mess, openly questioning the point of all this. He wouldn't have been wrong, but like many religious and family traditions, gathering on Yom Kippur to eat brisket off the good china was just something we did. It was about honoring the tradition, keeping the knot that held us together tied tightly. It was about reminding ourselves how to tie that knot, over and over again. I wasn't sure if our little family of four was going to be able to make it to the natural end of the evening. I couldn't be certain how much longer I could keep up the mental energy necessary to hide Daniel's breakdown. If I moved the conversation along, distracted the kids, and helped to get dinner on the table fast enough, we might make it to dessert.

We moved to the table set with green cloth napkins, a cream-colored tablecloth, and orange and yellow fall flowers placed in small glass vases in a single row down the middle. Daniel's father assumed the seat at one head, his mother at the other. Joe kept a watchful eye on Daniel, frequently squeezing his shoulder when he got up to get more water, intentionally catching his eye and smiling at him. Daniel was too important to him, and to ignore his son's pain was to pretend otherwise.

"This is delicious," I told my mother-in-law. "I honestly don't like brisket, but this is great!"

She had served brisket every Erev Yom Kippur that I had known Daniel. Why had I chosen this night to tell her I didn't like the meat? Maybe something in me was twitching, angry that I was wearing the veil, pretending Daniel was fine or that this dinner was purposeful and all was well.

"You don't like brisket? I wouldn't have served it!" She looked up at me with an amused look of astonishment.

"I don't like the meat," Julia announced next. She was chewing and chewing, and I knew it was only a matter of seconds before she spat out the whole gray wad onto her plate. I reached across the table, a napkin in my hand, ready to receive the contents of her mouth.

"Well," Daniel's sister said, "I love Mum's brisket. In fact," she turned to face Julia, "I'm going to make it for your birthday, Julia!"

"Noooo!" Julia cried out, but she was grinning because she loved her aunt. "Make me chocolate birthday cake with chocolate ice cream!"

Daniel remained fixed in his chair. His eyes followed the conversation, but he did not smile or talk. Looking back, Daniel's sister must have noticed something was terribly wrong with her brother, but she did not say anything. We all just carried on, like we were playing a big game of hide-and-seek. Daniel had found such a good hiding place, we could not find him. We didn't tell him we had given up.

James and Julia didn't seem fazed by Daniel's depleted affect that night, but maybe they had learned all too young how to rearrange what was in front of them to make it appear a different way. When it was time to leave, I wrestled James and Julia into their coats like one might stuff pillows into pillowcases. My mother-in-law packed up a brown paper bag with leftovers and handed it to Daniel to carry to the car. He took it from her while she leaned down to hug James and Julia. We stood at the door, and when Daniel reached up to hug his mother goodbye, he sobbed silently. My husband was in pain, and his mother loved him, but she didn't know how to help him. She could only wrap her arms around his body in a futile attempt to comfort him, as if kisses and hugs could wash the darkness from his mind. Joe hugged Daniel and whispered something in his ear that made Daniel smile, despite the tears leaking from his eyes.

With his round brown eyes, James stared up at Daniel. I waited for him to blurt out, "Why is Daddy crying?" But he never did. Maybe he knew better than to draw attention to Daniel's sadness. Maybe by the tender age of six, James understood the family code, the one my father had managed to pass down through the generations. We had all been taught well.

We walked out the door. James and Julia raced down the carpeted hallway. James tugged on Julia's shirt to hold her back, while Julia shrieked, "He's cheating! I want a redo!"

Once at the elevator door, James instructed her, "I'm pushing the elevator button, Julia."

"No! I get to push the button. He did the knocker!"

"She's right, James," I told him. "Julia gets to push the button; you got to bang the knocker."

"Fine," James mumbled and rolled his eyes. I got a glimpse of what he would look like in ten years, only in ten years, he would be bigger, taller, and stronger than I was, the stakes would be much higher, and we wouldn't be talking about pushing elevator buttons and banging door knockers.

Daniel stared straight ahead, focused on the dimly lit, red button. I remember being struck by how life spun around him like a whirlpool but did not pull him in. My family walked through the lobby and out the sliding doors of the ten-story building. Outside, the promise of night and silence greeted us. James and Julia climbed into their car seats, and I buckled them. Daniel opened the driver's side door and sat behind the wheel. I would have driven us home under the circumstances, but he probably didn't want James and Julia to think anything was out of the ordinary. Daddy is fine and will drive us home. I have a clear memory of this night, sitting in the passenger seat of the car, my husband steering the blue Volvo down the long, winding hill. The kids in their car seats in the back appeared oblivious to the tension and sadness hovering in the air, like a thick fog that we were all trying to make our way through.

I remember turning around and looking at them, chattering with each other, giggling in their private world back there. They tossed a stuffed zebra between the car seats. I glanced at my husband, his eyes staring straight ahead, weeping, while the rest of the world slid past him outside the car window. Covered by the darkness of the car, he didn't have to hide anymore. I too felt relief, like air being slowly let out of a balloon, like the worst, at least for this evening, was over. In the bubble that was our immediate family, I thought I could control what my children saw and how they interpreted it. My father had instilled in me the dangerous ability to go numb, to move on in the midst of suffering. I believed I had control over my children. I believed I could protect my husband. I believed I could make it all better.

It was a lesson I would have to unlearn. That night, I hustled James and Julia off to bed without mentioning why Daddy was weeping, why he did not come into their room or kiss them goodnight. I pulled their small feet through the legs of soft cotton pajamas, filled plastic sippy cups with water and placed them within reach on their night tables, and picked up sharp squares of LEGOs and tiny plastic animals from their wood floors. I could already picture the morning: I'd wake James and Julia, double down on my smile, let them wear whatever clashing outfits they pulled from their drawers, and pour them bowls of Lucky Charms while I waited for my husband's lithium to blessedly kick in.

THE SIN OF COMMISSION

I do not fast every Yom Kippur anymore. Nor do my husband and I have dinner at his mother's house the night before. But every year on Yom Kippur, I think about that evening at my in-laws' house, where I was so busy hiding Daniel's depression that I didn't realize my own sin of commission: denying that mental illness had a seat at our family table. I was too busy being the impeccable girl in my father's house, the one who raised perfect children. I couldn't see that mental illness was going to be a blinding flash for us, one that forever tainted my image of my own family. It would be years before I learned to look at that picture and still find beauty, not despite the mental illness but because of it.

NATURE QUEST WILDERNESS THERAPY

SOMEWHERE IN SOUTHERN UTAH, JANUARY 10, 2012

My parents are happily married, however having a bipolar father, my parents tend to yell and argue a fair amount. I am closer with my mom because she tends to give less punishments, whereas my dad is more stern and grounded. I have two siblings, an 11-year-old brother named Nathan, and a 17-year-old sister, named Julia. My little brother and I have a love/hate relationship with my sister. We enjoy teasing her out of love. My brother and sister have anxiety issues like me, which causes them to freak out whenever there is a family conflict.

ADMISSION

My memory of my relationship with Daniel is different from how James remembers it. I remember when James was young, I didn't argue enough with Daniel. I remember I had parenting issues I wanted to address with him, but I never confronted him with any of it. As far as I can remember, we had no conflict. We buried it all. We covered our disagreements with sideways glances, silent but knowing embraces, and unspoken deals that whispered, "I won't be angry if you forgive me." If Daniel and I had argued in front of the kids, maybe they might be more comfortable today with raised voices and criticism.

Now I have a new critic. James watches me and challenges me about whose truth I am writing here on this page. He is accurate in remembering that he was, in many ways, closer to me than he was to Daniel growing up. James went to me more often because I was around and probably because of my tendency to say yes, while Daniel had the ability to make a boundary and say no. James's description of his relationship with his siblings seems about right to me, ganging up with his little brother to tease Julia. He remembers yelling and arguing in our family, while I have no memory of that. Did I forget the fighting? Bury it? Is fighting part of what I need to reclaim and point the light toward? I honestly wish it were that easy. I'm telling you, reader, I would be relieved to admit to you that I tucked away the memory of family fights, marital spats, and sibling rivalry and that in coming to terms with those arguments, I was able to come to terms with James's mental illness. But that would not be true. I don't remember fighting with Daniel, and I don't remember loud family arguments because that kind of emotion did not pour out of me in the early years of my marriage. Like my father before me, my goal was to keep moving, to keep the peace, to avoid conflict like a preventable disease.

My children grew up in the same glass bubble I did. I know because I built theirs for them.

SILENT SCREAM

JANUARY 2001

In the winter of 2001, my mother was dying, but no one in my family believed her. When she complained, at the age of seventy-two, of leg pain, confusion, and fatigue, we carted her off to a geriatric psychiatrist. She had been diagnosed with heart disease and vascular disease, but her doctors insisted both conditions were under control through diet and medication. She would surely die of something else first. At least that's what my family was told. My mother called my sister one day at 3:00 a.m. and asked her why she wasn't awake and getting ready for work. She woke up at odd hours of the night, took a shower, dressed for the day, and poured herself some orange juice. But she also continued to be chic and elegant. She applied makeup to perfection and had a head full of silver-gray curls other women paid good money to imitate. She had lunch dates with friends and played a bridge game once a week.

Despite my mother's obvious but quiet unraveling, my father's work routine never shifted. He left their home in midtown Baltimore at 7:00 a.m. for the Abell Foundation downtown, where he researched and wrote grants after retiring from the *Baltimore Sun*. He returned from work at 6:00 for dinner. "I think she's fine," he told my sister, brother, and me whenever we asked him about her. We took my mother to psychiatrists, and behind closed doors, we told each other she was "losing it."

One day, I visited my mother at my parents' condominium, and I found her in her bedroom, still under the covers at lunchtime.

"Judy, I think I'm dying," I remember she said to me.

"She's not dying," my sister reassured me on the phone later in the evening. "She gets up every day, puts clothes on, goes shopping with her friends, and then likes to tell us she's dying. She's not dying. She wants attention from us."

About two months later, she crawled into her bed one last time and refused to get out. We took her to Union Memorial Hospital, where she was admitted for further testing. For days, my father, brother, sister, and I stood by her bed, wandered the halls of the cardiac care unit, ate dinners at an Indian restaurant a few blocks from the hospital, and waited for a diagnosis.

After my mother had been at Union Memorial Hospital for a week, a doctor delivered the news to us. We sat in rounded, white, plastic chairs in the waiting room of the floor. A muted television hung from a corner of the ceiling. "I think this is terminal," a young doctor in blue scrubs told my family. "There is really nothing more we can do. Her organs aren't receiving enough oxygen or blood because of advanced vascular disease. I would recommend hospice. I would say she may have a month to live."

At first, no one in my family believed the doctor. My father argued with him and told him she had recently been scanned for cancer by the best doctors at Johns Hopkins Hospital. He told this doctor she was on medication for vascular disease, took blood thinners and heart medicine; she had taken the drugs for years. Other doctors had assured her it was not getting any worse. How could this be? My father pressed the doctor before him, like the insistent journalist he was, determined to get this guy to come around to telling him the ending he needed to hear.

"Put her back in Hopkins," my father said. "I want her transferred to Hopkins."

"You have the right to move your wife wherever and whenever you want, Mr. Sandler," the doctor in the blue scrubs said. "But in my opinion, her condition is terminal. You will cause her unnecessary suffering by having her undergo further testing."

I will never forget the look on my mother's face when we told her she was being moved to Stella Maris Hospice Care. There had been some debate as to whether or not to tell her. She did not seem to be conscious much of the time, but she did have periods of time when she was lucid. If my sister held up a Garnet Hill catalog and my mother's eyes were open, she pointed to shoes or sheets she liked. Yes, we decided, we needed to tell her.

"Mom," I said to her as she lay on the hospital bed with her eyes closed, her silver curls falling around the pillow. She turned her head and looked at me. She knew who I was.

"We're going to move you from this hospital to Stella Maris. They can take better care of you there. Daddy and we think it's the best thing for you, okay?"

Now I realize that my mother, even in death, was not allowed the dignity of suffering aloud. She tried, in the only way she knew how to warn us she was running out of time. Something was happening inside her body, something invisible, much like I would witness in my son James many years later. She couldn't point to it or diagnose it, but it was there.

My father had created a world where retreat was shameful, and rest was discouraged for fear one would fall behind. Fall behind what? Of that, my siblings and I were never sure, but we all lived in fear of not being first, or at least of not being in the pack.

My mother lay in her hospital bed and opened her mouth, but she could not or did not speak. Her blue eyes, now a watery gray, also opened wide. Her mouth contorted. Her expression, terror. She understood she was going into hospice care. She looked like the face on Edvard Munch's *The Scream*.

What I think now is that it wasn't that we hadn't heard my mother or tried to recognize her pain. It was just that we didn't know how to stop long enough to feel it.

APOLOGY

When my brother and sister and I were old enough to read, but young enough to believe "Poetry Hour" might be a fun time, my father would gather the three of us on the sofa in the den, which was lined with floor-to-ceiling bookcases. A round, braided rug covered most of the brown-speckled tile floor that my mother called "cork." Sometimes, while my father walked around the room, he read us a poem, after which we were free to go. Other times, he asked us each to bring a favorite poem with us to read aloud. He sat on the rocking chair across from the sofa, staring intently at us, his arms leaning against his knees, while we read our poems to him. I liked Poetry Hour, probably because I was the youngest child and didn't have much better to do, but Poetry Hour kept my brother and sister away from their rooms, friends, and the telephone. I also loved capturing my father's full attention and scanning the titles of the books lined up on the shelves. It was at Poetry Hour that I first heard my father read poetic greats such as Ernest Thayer's "Casey at the Bat," and "Keep A-Goin'," by Frank Stanton, which had the unforgettable lines: "Ef you strike a thorn or rose, Keep a-goin'! Ef it hails or if it snows, Keep a-goin'! T'ain't no use to sit an' whine when the fish ain't on your line; Bait yer hook and keep a-tryin'—Keep a-goin'! . . . When you tumble from the top, Keep a-goin'! S'pose you're out of every dime, Bein' so ain't any crime; Tell the world you're feelin' prime—Keep a-goin'!"

My father liked "Keep A-Goin'," but I have come to resent the message of Stanton's poem. When I hear it in my head, I remind myself it's okay to sometimes *not* keep a-goin'. I believe my father meant well in teaching my siblings and me the poem. He wanted to instill in his children determination, drive, and resilience. I can't argue with those qualities in a person. But I wonder now if it is possible that a person can "keep a-goin'" to a fault?

I ran this inner conflict by my therapist. He pointed out that these traits of determination and endurance were necessary and helpful to my father and his ancestors, who survived the Holocaust, years of forced immigration, and religious intolerance. My father lived through the Depression and was a navigator on a ship during World War II. Surely, my therapist told me, "keep a-goin'" allowed him to survive difficult times. But is it possible, I questioned my therapist, in my father's determination to raise successful and accomplished children, he inadvertently but relentlessly taught us how to avoid conflict too well? Did he pave over the potholes instead of allowing us to feel the bumps, showing us how to make it to the proverbial top without stopping to wonder what that even meant and what we had to sacrifice in the process of getting there?

"It sounds like you have an apology in you," my therapist said to me in his light-filled office. He would wait in the silence that proceeded as long as I allowed it to last. I looked out the window of his seventh-floor office and stared at the tops of other buildings, some tree branches, and the roofs of restaurants.

"I might. I might want to apologize to James for not being able to stop myself, so there was no way I could stop him."

The therapist asked me what else I would apologize to him for.

I said, "I would apologize to him for all the times I could have suggested he take some time just to figure out what it was he was looking for. I would tell him, 'I'm sorry James. I couldn't pull you off the track. It wasn't in my DNA. I couldn't pull myself off the track.'" I was still looking out the window as I said these words. Then, I found it in me to catch the therapist's eyes. He was nodding slowly, and I joined him. A tiny, closed-mouth smile formed from the corner of my mouth.

FROM JAMES'S APPLICATION TO COMPASS ROSE

A Therapeutic Healing Community
"Offering a Choice for Adults to Recover from Debilitating and Traumatic Life Changes with Minimal Use of Mind-Altering Psychotropic Medication"

JULY 14, 2020

It was around this time that my mom's friend was looking for a person for a cultural exchange with a Parisian family. At 13, I flew to France by myself to meet the Picard's and was going to meet Olivier at the airport, someone who I had never met before. I had always been a crier and often have felt abandoned and this was one of those times where I was paralyzed in fear and crying while waiting in the Paris Charles de Gaulle Airport. Olivier brought me to meet his brother, Henri, who was my cultural immersion friend. Henri and I spent our time seeing the sights while drinking, smoking shisha, smoking marijuana, and camping out in internet cafes to play video games like World of

Warcraft, Counterstrike, and other competitive multiplayer online games. I was introduced to a new sense of independence and ability to navigate the metro by myself as I had been very dependent on my parents and others for a sense of direction.

BON VOYAGE

JUNE 2003

"Be good," I said as James and I waited outside the red velvet ropes of the security line in the international terminal at Baltimore/ Washington International Airport. "Have an amazing time. Enjoy everything, and talk French!"

I remember I wasn't teary or sad he was leaving. I felt proud that I had a son who, at thirteen years old, was responsible enough to fly by himself to France. Daniel and I offered to fly with him, but he told us, "Nah, I can do it. I'll be fine." And we had every reason to believe him.

Without looking directly at me, he said, "I'll call you, Mom. I'll call you when I get there. Or Mrs. Picard will call you, okay? I love you." He leaned down and wrapped his arms around me. I reached up and placed my arms around his narrow waist, kissing his cheek. He smelled like soap, and everything about him felt smooth and cool.

I stood there in the airport between throngs of people, their necks stretched, eyes searching for their person, hands waving goodbye. I saw James's back join the end of the security line. I had seen a lot of James's back in those years. The back of his black puffy coat cutting across a snow-packed mountain on his snowboard. The back of his red-and-white Friends School practice jersey, number twelve, trotting off to soccer practice. I watched his back from the driver's seat as he sauntered, in the direction of his pack, across movie theater parking lots. Sometimes, I waited an extra second after dropping him off at school to watch his backpack become one of many as he walked down the concrete path toward the middle school building. Now, I watched him load that backpack onto the conveyer belt and hold up his arms inside the body scanner. I followed his back as he collected his backpack and laptop on the other end of the security line, my eyes straining to keep up with his pace until his brown hair and navy blue T-shirt became one with everyone else.

He never once turned around and looked back at me.

DON'T BE LIKE ME

SEPTEMBER 1968

My adoration for my mother was profound, and the bond I felt with her was unbreakable. When I was a child, she was not ill; in fact, she was quite healthy. She smelled like Jean Naté body wash. I found her beautiful and funny, wise and calming. It was not unusual for my mother and me to go fishing on a Saturday afternoon in August at Lake Roland or Loch Raven, nearby reservoirs. She took me shopping at Bacharach-Raisin, a sporting goods store outside Baltimore, where I would survey the lacrosse sticks or buy some new cleats. I begged to go to the grocery store with her, where I could always talk her into buying me a Pez dispenser or giving me a quarter for the gumball machines outside the store. I didn't care how long we drove around in her blue Volvo station wagon. I felt like I was the best version of myself when I was near her.

The problem came when I had to go to school. I attended Mt. Washington Elementary in a tree-lined, old neighborhood in Baltimore City. The school was a four-story, light-brick structure with windows that stretched across the building, one row for each floor. The doors were heavy, green metal, impossible for a small child entering first grade to pull open. Most of the children in my neighborhood took the yellow school bus to school. All I had to do to get on this bus was walk out the front door of my house, turn right, and head down a hill, still within sight of my house and my mother the whole time. But I refused to take the bus to school.

For most of my first-grade year, my mother drove me the short ten minutes, then expected me to exit the car at the curb, just outside the building. I knew that if we arrived at school before 8:00 a.m., I would have to wait with swarms of other children inside the fenced playground area until the bell rang, signaling we were allowed to enter the building. This scene terrified me. I didn't want the fifth graders to glance over and see me crying for my mother as they whipped red rubber balls at each other, the boys huddled together like packs of wolves. So I made sure my mother and I arrived after 8:00 a.m.

My mother pulled our blue Volvo wagon up to the curb in front of the school. "Go ahead," she told me. "Once you get into your classroom and see Mrs. Lippins and your friends, you'll be fine. Now go on and be a big girl."

I watched the shapes my breath made on the window as I exhaled, wiped them away with my sleeve, and tried again. I could feel my mother's blue eyes staring at my back. I'm sure her head was tilted in a sympathetic way, but her hands gripped the steering wheel at ten and two like she was about to rip it from the steering column. I wanted to be a big girl. I yearned to be like all the other kids, carefree and laughing, running through those doors without their mothers. I took a deep breath and gathered my book bag and lunch box in my small, clenched hands. I pulled up on the plastic lock on the car door that looked like a shiny, green playing piece from my board game Sorry. I pulled up on the silver handle of the car door and glanced sideways at my mother, who was looking at me with enthusiasm, her eyebrows raised, her short, brown hair immobile on her head as she nodded encouragement.

"I can't do it!" I yelled. "I don't want to go to school! Take me home. Please take me home, I have a stomachache!" I wrapped my arms around my mother like some kind of baby animal. I saved these tantrums for my mother, with whom it was safe to completely unravel like this. I became almost feral with her, undoing all the rules my father enforced at home that advised me to get my act together, stop crying, and hold my head high. In the car with my mother, I tossed all that out the window and felt big feelings.

I was a thin, scrawny kid with brown, chin-length hair and cheeks that were now a splotchy mess. My mother was five feet eight, and even in the first grade, I sensed she was cool for a mom in the 1970s. But at this moment, her pink lipstick was doing nothing to soften her expression. Her thin lips were drawn tightly together in a straight line. She pried my arms from around her waist, climbed out of the driver's seat, walked around the front of the car, opened my passenger door, and said, "Enough of this nonsense. You're going to school. Stop crying and let's go."

Through the car window, I could see packs of children hurrying, pushing, and laughing their way through those green metal doors. Every one of them seemed just fine, more than surviving, possibly thriving without their mothers for the entire day. Did they not understand the risk involved in being separated from their mothers?

Mine reached into the car, her arms like octopus tentacles, grabbed my sweaty hand firmly in hers, and yanked my body out of the car. I allowed her to half drag me down the hallway, my two steps to every one of her long-legged strides. Peering into my classroom, I watched as my classmates stuffed their coats into wooden cubbies, watered the plants, fed the class fish, and returned books to the library. I had a class job, too, which was to take the attendance slip to the office, but since I was going home with my mother, I wasn't worried about it.

No amount of warmth radiating from my classroom could steal me from my mother. I squeezed her hand with renewed determination. Mrs. Lippins, an older woman with bleached hair the color and texture of straw, who had been teaching first grade twice as long as I had been alive, noticed us standing at the door—my mother's desperate expression and my hot, wet face. Rising from her desk, she tapped in her navy pumps across the room. In one imperceptible exchange, she and my mother traded places, and my hand was now gripping the cool, plump fingers of Mrs. Lippins.

"Have a good day!" Mrs. Lippins told my mother and shut the blonde, wood door to our classroom.

I heard my mother's shoes tap, tap, tap down the linoleum hallway, away from my classroom. Mrs. Lippins let go of my hand and walked back across the classroom. She called the class over to the rug and sat down in her rocking chair. My face remained pressed against the block of glass in our classroom door. First graders are empathetic little people, and I think my classmates were probably frightened as I wept, banged my fists against the door, and attempted to see one last glimpse of my mother through the thick, blurry window.

NURTURE

It is possible I pushed James into the shark tank before he could swim. We sat in Gymboree classes together when he could barely walk, and when he finally did walk, I couldn't wait to sign him up for kiddie soccer. It wasn't so much exposing James to all the activities that I regret; it was the expectation that he would go with enthusiasm and run eagerly away from me toward the very crowd of children whom I used to fear.

I felt great pride when James hurried into his kindergarten class, his soccer practice, or his gymnastics lessons. Because I had grown up embarrassed about the part of myself that suffered from separation anxiety, I desperately wanted James to be independent, to function with confidence away from me. Perhaps I taught James how to go numb and how not to feel, as my father had successfully taught me. I don't remember James ever turning to me and saying, "I am not going to school," or, "I don't want to go to soccer." Maybe he knew I didn't want to hear it; I expected of him an ease with people and groups that I never had at his age. Maybe he sensed I would have forced him to go anyway. This possibility is one I regret because he was probably right. Maybe he learned at a young age, as did I, that screaming, crying, and feeling something weren't worth the pain. Feelings did not breed sympathy. Fear was met with a harder push from my father toward whatever it was I feared.

So set was I on having a perfect family and keeping James from failing in any way—so determined was I to prevent him from experiencing the shame and embarrassment of the separation I felt as a child—I am afraid I drowned out his ability to say, "Help. Please help me."

PHONE CALL TO PARIS, FRANCE

JUNE 2003

James had been in France for a week, but I had not heard from him or from his host mother, Anna Picard. I was more curious than worried. I knew Anna worked as an urban planner in Paris and her husband, Emile, at an investment firm. It was a Sunday morning in June when I finally decided to call, 10:00 Baltimore time, 4:00 in the afternoon in Paris.

"Hi, Anna? This is Judy Sandler in the States." I paced around our small kitchen in Baltimore. The few times I had spoken to Anna on the phone before James left for his trip, she seemed like someone I'd known for much longer. What I needed to hear now was that all was well in Paris, that James and Anna's son, Henri, were seeing the sights, and that James was speaking French like a native.

"Judy? Yes! Hello! How are you? Everything is wonderful here. So good of you to call!"

"Well, James said he might call when he arrived, but since I didn't hear anything, I thought I would give you a call. How's it going? How are the boys?" I wanted to hear her tell me what an outstanding kid James was—helpful, kind, and open to trying everything they offered him. I needed to hear that he was not missing me. I could hear my father's voice inside my head: "He's great, Jude! What a kid, look at him now!"

She didn't fail me.

"Oh, James is lovely! What a great boy and so polite. Yes, Henri and his best friend, Martin, are showing James a wonderful time in Paris. They are like a pack of brothers, you know? They get along so well. It's hard to imagine they had not met until last week." Anna's English was nearly perfect, considerably better than my French. She spoke with a lovely accent.

Hearing Anna say the exact words I wished her to say allowed me to exhale, and I felt my body melt just a little. "That's great to hear. I'm relieved he's having fun and they're getting along so well. I hope he's behaving and offering to help you sometimes."

James had given us no reason to believe that he would be anything but enthusiastic, charming, and fun while he was at their house. But something in a hollow part of my stomach, a fluttering in my brain, wouldn't let me believe all was well with James in Paris. Maybe because I knew all too well that at James's age, I would have been a puddle on the floor of their kitchen, pathetically attached to my mother on the phone. Or maybe the memory of Daniel's bipolar episode, although it had been over five years ago by then, was palpable enough in my mind that the suddenness of it, how quickly it darkened our days, had me wondering if James would be happy and safe, wherever he was in the world.

"Ahhh, yes! He is much better behaved than Henri. You know, he loves to eat, your son. He loves the French cheese, the bread, and the wine!"

Wine? Did she say wine? Maybe James was learning about the art of fine French wines. I was okay with that. Maybe. He was only thirteen years old.

"Wine? That's great, I guess. Well, I don't want to keep you. I just wanted to check in and make sure James had arrived and that all is well. We can't wait to meet Henri and have him stay with us in August."

Daniel and I had already planned a trip to Washington, DC, with James and Henri when they got here, plus a few days at Rehoboth Beach in Delaware. Henri, we later learned, was well traveled and had been to Africa, toured all over Europe, and spent summers in a family home in Provence. Rehoboth Beach had nothing on Henri.

"Yes! Yes! Henri is excited about being with James in Baltimore and says you will take him to the beach. He will love that. Henri loves the ocean. Next summer, we want to take the boys to Corsica. James will love it there."

"Corsica? That would be amazing. James has definitely never been to Corsica. Thank you so much for having him and also for the invitation to Corsica. That's fantastic. Tell Emile we said hello, and please tell James to be good and that we miss him!"

There are multiple ways our children slip a little from our parental grasp, and it's true, there is no one card in the deck I can flip over and say, this is the one. But looking back, this trip to Paris, this extravagant invitation to Corsica, my thirteen-year-old son enjoying wine—maybe I was too easily swayed that this was all a good thing for James. Maybe I heard what I wanted to hear, and the riskier the better. I think I was secretly pleased to hear James was the risk-taker I never was, that he didn't have a problem having fun and making friends away from home. I found a quiet pride in discovering he was not me, after all.

I glanced out our kitchen window. It was so humid outside that drops of water clung to the windows. I saw our bluestone patio, a small pond, and an acre of green but very dry grass in a field below. I wondered what Anna saw when she looked out her kitchen window from the eighth floor of their stone building. I imagined she watched small cars start and stop on crowded streets, maybe with people resting on wrought iron chairs at cafés that lined those streets. The views from our kitchen windows differed vastly, but I felt like Anna and I were more the same than we were different. I was wrong. I have learned now never to assume anything about how anyone parents. You never know what lies beneath a child's facade. Probably, Henri could be poked and triggered a hundred times and still remain a sleeping bear.

Not so for James.

"Okay, Judy. We will hug James for you. So good to talk to you! Do not worry about James. He is a good boy and practicing his French! Talk soon, au revoir!"

Anna barely waited for me to say goodbye before she hung up. I listened to the silence on the other end of the phone and became consumed by the feeling that my son was thousands of miles away from me. Too far. It was a feeling in my lower stomach, like a bottomless well.

Something was not quite right.

WHAT CAME BACK

JULY 2003

James walked toward us in the arrival terminal of Baltimore/ Washington International Airport, backpack slung over his right shoulder, fingers sweeping his long brown hair from his eyes. Gone were his loose athletic shorts and cotton T-shirt. Gone were his high-top tennis shoes with the laces intentionally untied. Three weeks had passed, and he appeared to have grown two inches and not gained a pound. This teenager approaching me was clothed in tight black jeans, despite the sweltering late July temperatures in Baltimore. A white leather belt with a silver buckle wrapped around his hips, and a black crew neck T-shirt hung off his shoulders. A brand-new pair of Adidas Country tennis shoes, white with green suede stripes, were tied tightly to his feet. I looked twice to make sure this man-child striding toward me was my son. It was James, just the French version.

Daniel and I bombarded him with questions as soon as we piled him and his suitcases into the car. "How's your French? Any better? Did you speak French mostly or English while you were there? How are Henri's brother and sister? Did you see a lot of them? What is the house like? What did you see in Paris? How are Emile and Anna?"

Our questions were met in the back seat with an eye roll, a deep sigh, and obfuscation. If we thought his outward appearance had changed, his attitude toward us had completely flipped. Gone was the enthusiastic, innocent, sparkly boy I had watched walk through security a month ago.

"You know," James said and probably rolled his eyes at us again, although we could not see him, "we went around."

And noncommittally a minute later, "The house is cool. It's not a *house*, it's a *flat*."

And, "Yeah, Henri's brother and sister were around sometimes. We hung with them."

And, "Anna and Emile are not like you. They're cool. They aren't, like, asking Henri a million questions all the time. We got to do stuff. Like go out at night and sleep late."

It was dark outside and very late. At some point, James closed his eyes and leaned his head back on the seat. Cool air blew through the vents, but it still felt warm in the car, and I was getting hotter. I glanced over at Daniel, hoping to communicate with him without the need for words: *Give me some sign, Daniel. Some sign that you understand this child is still our son, the one that chatters about his days, smiles often, loves school, his teachers, and his parents.* Daniel stared straight ahead at the highway. I wasn't sure he even saw me look over at him, pleading with my eyes for reassurance as we sped along the Baltimore Beltway in silence.

Hot, loud silence.

THE PERFECT STORM

When I'd left James at the airport three weeks earlier, I dropped off a naive boy who had inhaled one joint in his life and tried a beer, or maybe none. I'd left a kid who still didn't mind being around his parents. The James who came back was secretive, sullen, and he frequently asked to sleep over at a friend's house. But we sent him back to Paris and the Picards the next summer and the summer after that. Maybe Daniel and I were slow learners, or maybe we had no idea we were using a pitchfork to poke our bear when we thought we were using our finger.

What I know now is that over those three summers in France, James picked up a cigarette habit that followed him off and on for the next fifteen years of his life. He drank a lot of hard liquor, wine, and beer, danced in sweaty nightclubs, and stayed out until the small hours of the morning, when James and Henri would stumble back to the Picards' flat in the upscale, genteel Seventh Arrondissement, home to the Eiffel Tower and the Musée D'Orsay, with its impressionist art collection. James and Henri woke up wherever they'd passed out, ate chocolate croissants, baguettes, dried meats, and fine cheeses, washed it down with cold Orangina, and did it all again.

I have the luxury of hindsight now, and I think about it like this: A seemingly fearless preadolescent boy, eager for independence and good times, went to live for three weeks, for three consecutive summers, with a handsome French boy who already owned that independence and had mastered the art of fun.

From my perspective, it was the perfect storm.

I'M GLAD YOU ASKED

"Why, even with all of your misgivings and your son's new sullen attitude, did you allow him to go back to France for two more summers?"

Reader, I want to ask you a different question: Have you ever been in a car accident? Did you see it coming? Could you have predicted that before you got to where you were going, a car would pull out in front of you and you would slam into it? After the front end of your car smashed into itself, how many times would you utter the phrase, "I swear, I just didn't see that car"?

So I tell people if I had known he was genetically inclined to substance use disorder, had I been aware that mental illness ran through his DNA, maybe I would have tried harder to control who he hung out with, where he went. I'm not sure I could have attempted to control him anymore. He was a teenager. Teenagers go through things. Like a car that pulls out in front of you, I didn't see it coming.

ROSE-COLORED GLASSES THAT PRODUCE OPTICAL DELUSIONS

I don't blame Henri or the Picards for the fact that when James swigged his first shot and inhaled his first bong hit, his brain probably lit up in very different ways than Henri's did. By the time James left for college, he was addicted to these substances, but Henri was not. "In those who are pre-disposed to substance use disorder," says the National Institute on Drug Abuse, "early exposure to substances is linked to addiction."

Memory is a biased tool. My recollection of James as a boy, perched on the edge of the pool of adolescence, and his memory of that same boy seem to exist as two different pictures. Mine is glossy and printed in color. I remember him as eager, confident, and daredevilish. His memory is of a boy plagued by the worry of abandonment and fear. In his application to Compass Rose, a therapeutic community that claims to stabilize those with mental illness without the use of medication, he wrote that he "had always been a crier" and had "often felt abandoned." Going to live with the Picards in Paris, he said, "was one of those times where I was paralyzed in fear and crying while waiting in Paris Charles de Gaulle Airport."

About eight months after James was asked to leave Compass Rose because of behavior deemed "unacceptable to the community values," I spoke with him on the phone. "Would you, today," I asked him, "write the same thing about your memory of going to France to stay with Henri? Would you say you were paralyzed in fear at the airport until you found the Picards? Do you still feel like you are abandoned by Dad and me?"

"I don't know," he said. "I mean, it was scary. I was thirteen years old, and I guess I was scared."

"I remember you wanted to go to France," I told him. I don't know why I had become so fixated on this, but I was determined to figure out how our memories of this time could be so vastly different. I felt uncomfortable and sad about his accusation that we abandoned him. "Would you agree that you were eager to go and that you asked to do the exchange with Henri?"

"Yeah," James agreed. "I wanted to go, and I had a good time while I was there. It was just a feeling I remember at the airport. I was really scared until I saw them."

I didn't believe him. He was a kid who took risks without breaking down and usually succeeded at whatever he tried. I took real pleasure in watching him learn how to play the guitar, kick a soccer ball into the top right corner of the goal, and weave down a mountain on a snowboard. The question now seemed to be if *he* ever really took pleasure in learning those things. And at what cost?

Is it possible that in my attempt to keep the memory of James's childhood a neat and glossy one, one that matched my expectation of what a happy childhood should look like, I recreated the memory and forced it to match my own hopes and expectations for him? So eager was I to see James succeed in every aspect of life, I failed to stop him before he boarded that first plane to Paris, turn him around, look him in the eyes, and ask him if he was feeling overwhelmed. How would I have known if he felt abandoned? I never asked. I had done it again. I had passed the stain on to him.

His use of the words "abandoned" and "paralyzed in fear" to describe his trip to France made me snap to attention. It's like we both paid to see the same movie, but mine was seen through a rose-colored lens. That gangly boy running by me in the slow-motion reels of my mind will always be strong-willed and self-assured, fearing only what he couldn't immediately master, smiling, and moving toward something, never away. That boy was not abandoned in my mind.

Maybe I handed James the skeleton in my closet, the one that rattled behind me wherever I went: I could do better. I should be doing better. Maybe James too felt that skeleton creeping up on him.

HIT ME WITH A BRICK

MAY 2007

Because I never changed my name from Sandler to my husband's last name when I married, I managed to remain anonymous at Friends School of Baltimore. For my children, however, who shared my husband's last name, life at school was not as easy. Expectations loomed; James, Julia, and Nathan walked in tall shadows down those hallways. Daniel had graduated from Friends, as had his father, his sister, and his sister's husband. When we were dating after college, Daniel's mother liked to tell me the story of how embarrassing it was for her and Daniel's father when Daniel won the "Excellence In" award in math, French, *and* history. There exists today a scholarship at the high school, a vestibule in the performing arts building, and a fund established to bring visiting authors to the lower school—all in the name of our family. To make my children feel even more like they were swimming in a fishbowl, I taught in the lower school while they were students there.

In the spring of James's tenth-grade year, his biology teacher, Cindy Hall, emailed, saying she wanted to meet with me. Preferably in my classroom, she wrote, so James wouldn't see us together. "I'm free at 4:00 this afternoon," I emailed back to her. "James will be at lacrosse practice. Come over to my room."

Cindy walked into my third-grade classroom and looked perplexed. Small, blue plastic chairs sat tucked under the low, round tables. Motivational posters—"Everyone Is Welcome Here, Everyone Belongs" and "You Make a Difference"—plastered the walls. A long, green strip illustrating each letter of the cursive alphabet hung over the whiteboard at the front of the room.

"Have a seat," I said, motioning toward the adult swivel chair at my desk. Upper school teachers looked so awkward to me in my elementary school room.

"Oh, I'm fine," she said, sitting down in a blue plastic chair. "I love being in lower school classrooms. They're always such warm and happy places."

I had to agree with her. Little children, little problems. Big children, bigger problems. I joined her in a low plastic chair at the round table and began to worry about the purpose of this meeting. I looked at Cindy and raised my eyebrows. She had taught biology at Friends for more than twenty years; students loved her, and their parents trusted her.

"So, is James failing biology?"

"Oh no, it isn't that. He's doing great. You know, that kid is funny. If his grades were slipping, trust me, I would just talk to him. He listens to me. He loves biology."

Okay, I thought to myself. *Why is Cindy Hall sitting in my classroom after school if James is not failing biology?*

She took a deep breath. "Look, Judy, I'm here because I'm worried about James. I really like him. We have a close relationship. But I have to let you know that I'm concerned. I've seen him leave campus with his friends. They slip off at lunch, and sometimes again right before lacrosse practice. When he has biology in the afternoon, his eyes are bloodshot. He looks high, and he wreaks of marijuana."

My eyes narrowed, and I tilted my head. How could James be pulling this off in the middle of the day? Wouldn't someone have caught him by now?

"Wow," I said. "Thanks for letting me in on all of this. I'm wondering why no one has turned him in. Are you the only teacher or administrator who sees him leave campus?"

Cindy smiled, looked right at me with her hazel eyes, and shook her head. "No one wants to rat out your son."

She didn't have to say anything else. It was like turning the cardboard cylinder on a kaleidoscope and watching the tiny triangles settle into a design that my brain recognized: everybody knew, and no one was talking. The faculty understood that if they turned James in, he wasn't getting kicked out of the school, so what was the point?

Cindy was doing me a favor. She cared about my kid. I nodded slowly. Up until then, Daniel and I had viewed James's use of weed as an adolescent nuisance. But now he was leaving school, getting high, and returning to practice in an altered state. Daniel and I were going to have to confront James with a problem, not a growing pain.

I thanked Cindy for her time and for her genuine concern for James. I watched her walk out of my classroom, down the brightly lit hallway, past the lower school office, and out the single glass door of the old stone building. In some ways, that late afternoon marked the next chapter of my life. The chapter where I began to fight with James about how much pot he smoked, where I searched his room when he wasn't home, where I smelled his T-shirts before I threw them in the washing machine. In the years to come, it would sometimes feel like this is all we fought about.

I packed up my bag with a stack of spelling quizzes and a few black-and-white marble notebooks the kids used as personal journals, and I remember thinking how I wished I could spend the night in the quiet warmth of my third-grade classroom instead of going home to what I knew was going to be a long, loud, and ugly evening. Where was my Norman Rockwell family, each child returning home at the end of the day for dinner and homework? At that moment, it wasn't James's pot use I feared, it was telling Daniel and then having to confront James. I knew how my father would have handled this one. But Daniel didn't go for that style of discipline where we brushed the incident into the dustpan, tossed it in the trash can, and sat down to dinner.

I felt caught in between.

It's only now that I can see I was worrying about the wrong thing. It didn't matter how torn I felt between Daniel and James. I didn't need to feel comfortable. I needed to address James's desire to self-medicate all day long.

NATURE QUEST WILDERNESS THERAPY

SOMEWHERE IN SOUTHERN UTAH, JANUARY 2012

I've always been a super stressed and anxious person. I started self-medicating with pot to feel happy and buzzed. Depression and just lacking a purpose in life has been a problem recently when I've been struggling academically in school. The anxiety and depression have been more noticeable within the past three years than before. I tend to break down crying or get a lot of rage when I am worried or upset about anything. I used to be addicted to World of Warcraft in sophomore year of high school but switched over to drugs as a substitute. I've had a problem recently with spending too much money too quickly and living sustainably.

My parents and I have always disagreed upon what is an appropriate use of weed and how often it's okay to partake. This has created a lot of distrust between us in regard to communicating honestly and listening to my parents. I've always been stubborn and independent, always defying my parents' expectations whatever they may be. Whether it was playing three Varsity sports while smoking before practice and at lunch or maintaining a 3.0 GPA while goofing off. My parents have always had high expectations for my future. They haven't agreed with me on much of anything or have been proud of me since my senior year of high school when being accepted to college. My brother and sister have been able to learn from my mistakes and avoid my downfalls. This has made some distance between me and my brother and sister. This has kept me kind of alienated from my parents and has kept me from asking them for help when I have noticed problems in my life.

BEHIND CLOSED DOORS

MAY 2007

James sat down on the edge of his bed, as he'd been asked to do. Daniel remained standing while I paced back and forth at the end of the sleigh bed and ran my hand over the smooth, curved edge of the wood. I glanced at Daniel, expecting him to start this conversation. I knew what we had to do, but the room felt small, like there was not enough air in it for the three of us to breathe.

The moment reminded me of when James was little and in trouble for being unkind to his sister or running from his time-out chair. I was having trouble escaping the irony of all the memories in this room. His bed stood firmly in the middle of the room, made up with navy-and-white striped sheets, cotton blankets, and a red-and-white patchwork quilt. Athletic awards lined his bookcases and crowded the fireplace mantel, with red antique tins decorating the tops of his desk and dresser. The once innocuous tins advertised tobacco on the front in worn gold script, but I had found ziplock bags of weed hidden inside them. A blue rag rug covered most of the pine floor. Threads of the rug were loose from when James was younger and had run his Hot Wheels cars up and down the woven fabric, the tiny plastic tires tangling in the fibers. The rug also had water stains from when James and I used to clean out his large fish tank that now stood empty in the corner. There was a fireplace in the room, but I don't think he ever used it. Though at that point, I couldn't be sure I knew what James did or didn't do.

"James," Daniel finally said, "Mrs. Hall came to see Mom this afternoon at school and informed her that she has seen you leave campus with friends. She says that she believes you're getting high off campus and then returning to class and to practice. She told Mom that she has seen this happen many times." Daniel stared at James and waited for him to reply.

One dependable trait about our son has always been that he tells the truth when he is caught. He may withhold information, but when approached with a direct question, he doesn't lie. His hands were on his knees, and he stared at the ceiling. He sighed deeply with obvious disgust and disbelief, as if the sigh itself said, "Why are you even bothering me with this question?"

"Yes," he told us. He left campus with friends, and yes, they got high in the woods behind the Cathedral of Mary Our Queen, an enormous church next to Friends School on Charles Street. "The faculty is so stupid, Dad. They just let us go. We can totally just walk up Boxhill Lane, and Mr. Santos is standing there, out for his afternoon smoke, and he waves to us."

While James was busy blaming the faculty, Daniel and I tried to redirect the responsibility for his behavior back to him. But James was not having it.

"Yes," he told us again with a degree of confidence and assuredness that seemed shocking to me, "I get high in the middle of the day. I like it. It relaxes me. You and Dad have a glass of wine at night. Consider it my glass of wine."

I paced across the room at this point to lean on the fish tank. A loud sigh escaped from my chest. I felt afraid of this conflict and could not speak. I admit now that I didn't want to give James any kind of consequence for his behavior that would negatively affect his ability to attend lacrosse practice or keep up with his academic schedule. So instilled in me was the "keep a-goin'" mantra, that I feared if we punished James, if we grounded him or put into place some consequence for his actions, he would fall behind in his schoolwork or lose his starting position on the team. The snowball effect of what might have seemed like logical punishments for smoking pot every day rolled around in my brain.

I feared Daniel would take away lacrosse from James or tell him he was grounded for a month, thus trapping an angry bull in the proverbial china closet. It was easy for Daniel to order up the punishment, but he and I both knew I was the one who would be expected to carry out the sentence. Daniel worked late at the office and at home and traveled frequently for work. I already felt like I did not have enough power or control over James to play prison guard, and this is what scared me the most. I knew James deserved and needed boundaries, but James and I both knew that while I may have held the key, all he had to do was apologize and I would unlock the door. I was too afraid of letting him hurt, allowing him to fail.

I wish I could rewind this movie now; there's a lot I would undo. I can imagine it now, but I would have to rewind the movie from a place that does not begin here. I'd have to change the way I interacted with James long before this moment. Over and over again, I would have told him no: No, you can't go to Shenanigan's

Toy Store every day after school; no, you can't have another candy at 7-Eleven; no, you can't sleep out tonight; no, no, no. And then would he have developed a stronger sense of resilience? A way to self-soothe without marijuana? If I could go back, I might change the way I disciplined James, but how far back would I need to go? Where was the beginning?

"There is so much wrong with this argument, James," Daniel said, "I don't know where to begin." He leaned his hip against James's desk and looked directly at him. "You are not twenty-one. Therefore, you are not of legal age to drink. Marijuana is illegal in this state for anyone. And I don't drink in the middle of the day to relax. Maybe we need to be talking about what kind of stress you are experiencing and how we can help you deal with it without getting high. Because this is not an option for you anymore. Do you understand? In case I need to remind you, you aren't allowed off campus until your senior year, and you are never allowed to get high. Ever."

I could tell Daniel was trying to keep his voice down, but the "ever" came out between clenched teeth.

"Do you hear me, James?" Daniel said and made an obvious attempt to lower his head to James's level so he could look him directly in the eye.

"Thanks, Dad, for that information. Shit, all this time I thought we were allowed to get high at Friends School. Now you tell me we can't?" James had a smile on his face, as if he were actually amused by his own sarcasm.

I would not have blamed Daniel if he had shouted at James, stormed out of the room, or even gotten into James's face and stared him down. But I decided that rather than risk the further wrath of Daniel, it was time for me to step in.

"Don't get smart with us, James," I finally said. "We're trying to stay calm and help you find another way to deal with your stress at school. I think we should find someone for you to talk to—like a psychologist—about drug use. I'm feeling like we are at a turning point here, and we really don't want you kicked out of school."

"Like they are really going to kick me out of Friends after Gramps and Dad? I'm not getting kicked out of school, Mom." His head was tilted toward me, but his eyes looked elsewhere, as if this should have been obvious to me.

So James was aware that being a Sherman at Friends was a blessing and a curse. "Don't be so sure of that, James. You play by the same rules as everyone else at Friends," I told him, even though I had heard otherwise from Cindy Hall. "Forget about getting caught, forget about blaming other people. Will you agree to talk to someone who might be able to help you?" I asked him.

He stood up from the bed. Apparently, we were finished here. He ran his hand across the long bangs that hid his eyes. "Sure," he said quietly, "I'll talk to someone." He grabbed his laptop from his desk and walked out of his bedroom, down the hallway, to a spare bedroom where he liked to play *World of Warcraft*.

Daniel and I glanced at each other, unsure who had come out on top of that conversation. In a few seconds, I heard the familiar sound of blazing gunfire from the video game. James had placed the headphones on his ears and entered another world. "Get out, get out!" I heard him shout. "One shot! Oh my god, wipe." He had gone from one addiction to another.

I may have held the key, but I didn't know which room to lock him in. And I was too afraid to try.

HINDSIGHT IS HELL

What if, instead of offering to put James in therapy, we had pulled him from private school and enrolled him in public school? What if, instead of driving him to therapy sessions for a year and paying $200 for each appointment, we had taken him on a tour of the Baltimore City jail and had him talk to some of the inmates about the value of an education? Instead, I foolishly believed that after a few sessions with a good therapist, James would just get better; he would realize weed was not the answer.

In my snow-globe crystal ball, I saw the snowflakes settling in our little village. Daniel and I would pick James up with tweezers and glue him back to the bottom of the base, upright and stronger than before.

A CONVERSATION: BOYS WILL BE BOYS

MAY 2009

In the spring of James's junior year, the Manns' basement became the hangout of choice for James's pack. Sometimes, I got a call from him at midnight, letting me know that he was going to "just sleep at Mann's, okay?" I never understood why the Mann parents were unaware their basement was a den of bongs and beer. But by May of that year, I became convinced that if I directed Justin Mann's attention to the fact that there was a pack of boys in his basement getting wasted on a regular basis, he would consider putting an end to it.

It was a Sunday morning in 2009, after James had spent another night in the Manns' basement, that I decided to give Justin a call. "Hey, Justin," I said into the phone while I stood in my kitchen, scraping up bits of scrambled egg from the stove. "It's Judy Sandler, James's mother. How are you?"

"Judy Sandler! How's everything? I think James spent the night here last night. Great game he had on Tuesday. What a win!"

At least he knew James was in his house somewhere. "Yeah, that was a great game. I love watching this team play. There's chemistry between those boys. They've been playing together for so long now, they know where each other will be in a split second, you know? Could be a good season for them." I paused, knowing I needed to get to the point. "Justin, I'm calling because I'm concerned James and the boys are doing some serious partying in your basement. James is usually too drunk or high to drive home and calls us most Saturday nights to say he is spending the night at your house. I guess we're wondering if you know what is actually going on down there. We're concerned about James. Seems like every weekend, these boys are together, getting high."

There was an uncomfortable silence. I thought Justin hung up on me, but he finally spoke.

"You know, they *are* teenage *boys*," he said, placing emphasis on the words "are" and "boys," as if that was news to me and was supposed to make me feel better. As if the fact that they *are* teenage *boys* made it okay that my son was wasted in his basement. "If you want me to send James home, I can do that. But I assure you they're all fine."

"No, don't send him home," I said, panicked in that second that he would humiliate James by calling down to the basement and shouting that James's mother wanted him to come home now. My face flushed, and I added quickly, "I just wanted to make sure you knew what was going on. But it sounds like you do."

I should have been angry. I should have taken Justin up on his offer to send James home. Here was another person willing to blur the line between a partying kid and an addicted kid. Easy for

Justin to look the other way. He was no better than the teachers at Friends who pretended they didn't notice James leaving campus.

"Oh, we do!" Justin assured me, and if I could have seen him wink at me, I know he would have.

"Okay, Justin, you convinced me. Maybe just visit them down there occasionally and make sure they're alive?" I was only half kidding. It isn't that difficult to keep track of children, even when they are adolescents and seemingly out of parental control.

But the truth is, James's substance use was already out of my control. According to a statistic from American Addiction Centers, one in seven young adults will develop a substance use disorder. That one was my son. The problem was that I was not willing to rock James's boat and call him out on his problem. I had been so well trained to look the other way, ride out the wave, and flatten the conflict until it made only a bump in the road. Nothing too serious.

"You got it, Judy. On my way down there now. And when they look at me and ask what I am doing down there, I will tell James you requested the pleasure of my company."

That was fine with me. I didn't care that it seemed like Justin was throwing me under the bus or, at the least, playing passive-aggressive ball with me. It seemed the least he could do was walk downstairs.

"Thanks, Justin. See you Thursday at the next game?"

"Absolutely," he replied, as smooth as the smoke rings rising to the ceiling of his basement.

RED FLAGS AND STARS THAT DO NOT ALIGN

JUNE 2009

James's high school years were loud with warning bells involving pot or alcohol that all faded with time into a low, ringing sound that we talked ourselves into calling normal. One summer, near the end of eleventh grade, a few of James's good friends were invited to spend a weekend at a friend's beach house on the eastern shore of Delaware. James did not receive an invitation.

I remember he walked around the house that weekend sullen, angry, and especially unpleasant. "Why do you think you weren't invited to the beach?" I asked him on Saturday morning, trying to slay the elephant in the kitchen while he shoveled in spoonfuls of Raisin Bran at the table and I had a cup of coffee.

"I don't know," he mumbled between bites. "Maybe because Jack's mom is an idiot?"

"I doubt it," I said.

I felt badly he had not been included, but I also had a sense that there might be a reason. Though I never would have guessed the reason was that Jack's mother, Jennifer Pratt, knew James was buying, selling, and distributing marijuana, and she viewed him as a bad influence. I can't say I blamed her.

It was three years later on a cold, sunny afternoon in Roland Park that I shared with Jennifer that James had dropped out of Colorado College and was in a therapeutic wilderness program in the woods of southern Utah being treated for substance use disorder. I told her he'd called home in the middle of his sophomore year to let us know that he needed help. Jennifer said her husband was a regular at AA meetings at the Church of the Cathedral across the street from their house. He had been addicted to cocaine for many, many years. She said that she knew James was abusing weed in high school but never said anything to me because she felt it wasn't her story to tell. "It was James's story to share with you when he was ready."

I know now she was correct.

I wouldn't have listened to her. I was busy smudging a line that was incredibly easy to smear between facing the truth and looking away. It was pretty painless to look the other way. Real addiction lived out there in the land of other peoples' problems. Not mine. At the time, I chose to believe James was a "partying" adolescent, one safely ensconced in some bubble of privilege that would protect him as he sat in his private school classes, high as a kite, and drove his blue Toyota 4Runner just sober enough to smile and nod when a cop stopped him for a burned-out headlight.

It was easy for me to keep moving the line of addiction. It turns out other people helped me to blur the line. Jack's mother moved it when she didn't think it was her place to inform me of James's drug use. Justin Mann moved it because, well, "They *are* teenage *boys*." James's soccer coach moved it for me when he told me, "You can't teach that kind of aggression. If I could bottle it and sell it, I'd have winning teams every year." James's teachers moved it by not reporting him when they watched him leave campus.

What I didn't know about addiction hurt me. What I refused to see cost James and our family valuable time. We missed waving red flags. We didn't hear loud bells. There were stars, a trail of them, bad omens all, that made a menacing shape in the sky. It was easy to squint our eyes and claim we couldn't quite make out how they were aligning.

I look back now and wonder why I didn't call Justin Mann and ask him to tell James to get the hell out of his basement and come straight home. Or why we didn't just go and get him ourselves.

DR. BRAD SIGLER

APRIL 2008

Daniel and I sat in beige, fabric-covered chairs opposite each other. James sunk down on the brown leather sofa between us. Dr. Sigler was in his mid-fifties but looked a little younger in a blue button-down shirt and khaki pants with no belt. His wiry brown hair appeared to need a brush. From his swivel chair behind his desk, he focused only on James. "So, James, you have something you want to talk about with your parents?" It had been eighteen months of weekly therapy appointments. I expected to hear the sounds of progress: James had realized he was smoking too much and had planned with Dr. Sigler for alternative methods of relaxation.

"I guess so," James glanced up from his zone on the carpet and picked at his fingernails, which he did when he was nervous.

He looked at me, then at Daniel, his eyes resting again on the carpet in front of him. "What I want to tell you is that I like getting high. I mean, I know you disagree with me, but I don't think weed is dangerous in any way. It's a lot less addictive than alcohol. I have decent grades, I play three varsity sports, I'll go to college. Like, sitting in this office once a week isn't doing me any good. I don't want to talk to a therapist anymore. I'm not going to stop smoking weed. I like it."

A deep silence settled over the office. I stared out a smeary window at a tree in a patch of grass next to another office building. Cars steadily moved down York Road. I held my breath.

Dr. Sigler wasn't finished with us. I looked back at him. "I honestly think," he said turning his head from Daniel to me, "the best thing we can do for James at this point is to keep him safe. He has decided pot is his hobby, and he is going to continue to smoke with his friends. There isn't much point in my seeing James anymore if the goal of the therapy is to encourage him to stop getting high. I'm taking your money and not making progress with that goal. James is an honest, sincere, bright kid. He is set on his desire to use marijuana. I'm not sure what else I can do for him, or for you." Dr. Sigler's eyes peered out from behind silver wire-rimmed glasses.

I forced my body to be still and to consider what Dr. Sigler had just told us. So intent was my belief that I could control James's substance use, Dr. Sigler's words came at me like a dare.

And I always take a dare.

DO THEY COME PREASSEMBLED?

For a long time, I blamed the messengers. But now I understand Dr. Sigler was correct; there was nothing he or any of us could have said or done to stop James from using weed. He wasn't ready to quit. He was already addicted.

Now I know, from stalking websites such as the National Institute on Drug Abuse, that addiction, more commonly referred to today as substance use disorder, is a complicated disease of the brain and body that involves obsessive and compulsive use of substances, despite social and health consequences. Addiction, I now know, affects the part of the brain responsible for motivation, learning, reward, judgment, and memory. According to American Addiction Centers' research, genetic risk factors may account for half of the likelihood that a person will develop a substance use disorder.

Medically speaking, by the time James left Dr. Sigler's office that day, determined to keep smoking pot, his brain chemicals had already begun to recognize THC as a pleasure-producing substance. James now set out to do whatever he had to do in order to reach that pleasure state again. And again, and again.

SCARS

SEPTEMBER 2010

Because it was 1:30 in the morning, and because I could have sworn James was home asleep in his bed, I almost didn't answer the call. But then I saw "Baltimore City Police Department" roll across my cell phone screen.

"Hello?" I breathed into the phone.

"Is this Judy Sandler?" It was a man's voice.

"It is."

Was this *the call*? I wondered. The one where they tell me James is in the hospital or jail, or worse, where they ask me to come identify the body?

"This is Officer O'Brian. I'm here with your son and his friend, Max. You're going to have to come get him. I could have taken him in for possession of marijuana, trespassing, and violating the curfew, but a pretty boy like this isn't going to last long in the Baltimore City jail tonight. How about you just come get him?

We'll wait for you at Linkwood Park by the swings. You know where that is, right?"

"I do. Be right there," I whispered into the phone. Daniel was awake next to me. I guess he could hear the cop through the phone.

"You want me to go with you?" he said, lying on his back, eyes closed, arms crossed over his chest, his body completely still. "No, never mind. If I see him, I'm going to kill him."

For the next few years, I would receive many of these calls. And now, years later, they are still in my body and won't go away. My body remembers each buzz of my cell phone, every awkward conversation. If I am honest, whenever the phone rings now, I hesitate to answer. My chest tightens, and my mind spins. The most unforeseen, sudden changes of direction can come at you in the flash of a phone call. They are embedded in my emotional memory like a gash. A cut that just won't scar over.

SCARS II

OCTOBER 2015

Another call about 5 years later interrupted a small Halloween party Daniel and I were enjoying at the home of the Chases, in northern Maine.

"Hi, Judy, It's Chris. Sorry to bother you, but I really need to check in with you about James. Do you have a minute?" I stood up from the dinner table and stepped away from the pumpkins and gourds lining the table, which had seemed so festive earlier in the evening. *I just need a minute,* I indicated, raising a finger in the air.

Outside, in the cool autumn air, I listened to James's friend Chris describe James's unusual behavior. He spoke of what I now realize were growing signs of James's paranoia. James slept a lot during the day, Chris said. He had accused Chris of stealing a pendant that Chris had given to James as a gift. James had no plans for finding a job. I was aware that James had been put on "administrative leave" from his job at Oceanside Hospital, where he had been working as a recreational therapist, but I had assumed incorrectly that he was looking for another job. Maybe I wasn't calling him frequently enough. Maybe I didn't want to know. If I didn't text or call James daily, he may or may not have checked in with me. And in this way, I could go about my days without digging too deeply into the truth of James's life. But I heard Chris's voice over the phone that night, and I had to answer him and, indirectly, myself. Chris was the alarm, and I would need to wake up.

I closed my eyes, sighed, nodded, and paced the front yard of our hosts' house while I listened.

After the call, I had to knock on the Chases' door to rejoin the party. My eyes darted around the table while I swirled my cold shepherd's pie.

I know this; it's a strange phenomenon that I have gotten used to. My body is in a social situation, one that just ten minutes ago may have been warm, entertaining, and comfortable, but then, in the time it takes a cell phone to buzz, I physically exist in the same room, but mentally, I am completely distracted, my mind now focused on what I need to do to help James. At this particular moment, I was no longer entertained by the crackling fire and the miniature pumpkins.

The other guests scraped the last of their chocolate mousse from their white ramekins. Oh, how I wanted to be them.

SCARS III

OCTOBER 2016

Another call. This one was while I was driving to work. I wouldn't have picked it up, but the caller ID read "Portland, Maine," and that was where James lived now. It was his girlfriend on the other end, telling me she was in the process of checking James into the psychiatric unit at St. Mark's Hospital in Lewiston, Maine. He hadn't changed his clothes in a few days, nor slept, she said, and he had been roaming around the streets of Portland, stopping people to let them know he was there to help them, no matter what they needed. He told them he had special powers to heal.

"You want to talk to him?" Jessica asked me as I pulled into the lower school parking lot and looked for an empty space. I had to be in my classroom, ready to go by 8:00 a.m.

"Sure," I said, my mouth tightening into a straight line, my eyes closing into a long blink. Out my window, children played on the blacktop playground and huddled in groups, waiting for the morning bell to ring. They chased each other around the swings, screaming with delight as they fell in a heap on the wet grass.

"I'm trying to help these people, Mom," James said, and if you didn't know he was delusional at the time, you would have thought he sounded sincere and sane. "There are so many of them. And where are the doctors? I'm thinking maybe I should go to medical school so I can really help people, you know?"

It was only 7:30 in the morning. James's voice brought my focus back. My heart twanged against my chest, and despite the overcast skies, I began sweating under my light jacket. I gathered my book bag, pocketbook, and the stack of black-and-white marbled spelling journals, which I had to return to my third graders, from the back of the car.

"Well," I said because there was nothing I could say to him from my car in the Friends School parking lot in Baltimore to give order to his thoughts as he waited in an emergency room at St. Mark's Hospital. "It's good of you to care so much about other people. And you have always wanted to help people. Call me in a little while, okay? Or have Jessica give me a call."

"Okay, Mom. I love you."

"Love you too, bud."

I knew I was preparing myself to take care of other people's children that day in a way that I could not take care of my own son. Soon, I would get out of the car and hug the children in my classroom, comfort them when their friends were mean to them, and cheer for them when they made a breakthrough in math. I would be with them for eight hours, and then this evening, I would return their parents' phone calls, put to rest their worries about their daughter's anxiety, their son's aggression. While my own son would stare at a white tile floor in a cold, hard plastic chair in a hospital waiting room. I felt terrible guilt as I slammed my car door shut; I wasn't flying to Maine to attempt to save James.

I almost dropped the stack of notebooks as I walked down the path to the lower school, thinking about how I would make it through this day, my body in my third-grade classroom with other peoples' children, my mind in the psychiatric ward of St. Mark's in Lewiston, Maine, with my own son. I had to go make copies of the multiplication practice sheets and write the science homework on the board.

Oh, and I almost forgot, it was Braydon's birthday, and his mother was sending in cupcakes.

SCARS IV

DECEMBER 2010

I have scars all over my body, obvious to anyone who is looking. My knees bear multiple scars in frightening shades of purple and dark pink from a lifetime of trips and falls while running along trails in the woods. Once, a pebble the size of a small pill, but not as smooth, lodged in my knee and had to be removed by a doctor. Most recently, I was running a trail along a river in Maryland, feeling confident and listening to music on headphones, when I tripped over a rock, or maybe it was a tree root. My face took the worst of it; a slight scar just under my nose marks where my upper teeth sliced through my lip. It happened in a split second, not long enough for my brain to register the pain. I only realized what had happened after I put my hand to my mouth and tasted the coppery blood.

My left shoulder is misshapen due to a skiing accident on a family vacation to Utah. I hit an unexpected bump and fell hard. People in the lift line glanced over at me, assuming it was nothing, I bet, because how could I hurt myself attempting to come to a standstill in a lift line? But two ski patrols witnessed my rapid face-down into the snow. I heard one of them say, "Ouch. That was not okay." I felt nauseous, and my left shoulder protruded at an unnatural angle.

One ski patrol kneeled down and slid his hand underneath the back of my down jacket. "Definitely separated the shoulder and maybe cracked the collarbone." He looked at his buddy and motioned his head toward the snowmobile.

I had seen people wrapped tightly in gray flannel blankets get carried off in these snowmobiles, only their head exposed to the cold air. I felt sorry for them, their vacations ruined, knee or ankle surgery scheduled for when they arrived back in their hometowns. Now I was wrapped in the gray flannel blanket, taking a ride to the nearest ski lodge, where an ambulance waited. Once in the emergency room, a competent and swift-moving orthopedist took over. She slid a needle into a vein in my left arm, hooked me up to an IV dripping propofol, and rendered me unconscious for about twenty minutes while she manipulated my shoulder back into place. The scar looks like a bone that found a new home.

But these physical scars pale compared to memories I have of James's phone calls, the muscle memory no one can see. What I tell myself is that he is not me and I am not him. Nor am I in control of him anymore. He grew inside me and passed through my body, but I can no longer find myself in him, and I am willing to believe he can't find himself in me.

COLLEGE FOR ME

1980

Every October, my father drove my mother, brother, sister, and me to Philadelphia for his college reunion at the University of Pennsylvania. "Let's go look at the bridge, Jude," my father would say at each of these reunions, walking with me down Locust Walk, past the bookstore, and over the arched footbridge that spans Thirty-Eighth Street. The bridge was constructed in 1971 but was rededicated in 1974 as the Class of '49 Bridge, in honor of their twenty-fifth reunion gift. The donors' names are listed on a plaque hanging from the railing of the bridge. "Find my name, Jude. Can you see it?" My father stood close behind me, staring down at the plaque.

He nodded and smiled when I placed my finger on his name.

"There it is, Dad. Gilbert Sandler. Right there on the plaque. Pretty cool." I ran my finger over the raised letters of his name. Back home in Baltimore, there was no escaping the Penn red and blue. Khaki hats, with a red-and-blue ribbon wound around the brims, were piled on the shelf in the coat closet. Penn coffee mugs stacked up in our kitchen cabinets; special articles from the *Penn Gazette* hung in my father's study, fading under the glass.

"One day, Jude," Dad said, "you'll walk to class and cross this bridge. You'll go to practice on Franklin Field, you'll cross this bridge, and you'll see my name every time." He nodded slowly and placed his hands on my shoulders, like a man who had just bought a new car and felt like he got a good deal. I know he meant it as a wish for me, but his plan felt more like a trap.

"I really don't suggest any of the Ivies, Mr. Sandler," my college guidance counselor said at our first meeting in the fall of my senior year of high school. "They are extremely competitive right now, and unless she has some interest from the lacrosse coach, or we can get some help from the alumni side of things, Judy's SAT scores are not where they need to be for the Ivies."

The counselor's name was Helene Reynolds, a pleasantly round woman with smooth skin and very short, dark hair. Despite the ridiculous pressure she must have been under working at a private school in Baltimore, Mrs. Reynolds nodded her head at my parents and smiled in her pale pink lipstick. I remember sitting silently between my parents in a large, wooden chair painted glossy black with a gold college insignia stamped on the top, where my head would have rested if I had been relaxed enough to do that.

Instead, I sat on the edge of the chair, my hands clenching both sides of the seat, because I knew how important this meeting was to my father. I listened to Mrs. Reynolds rattle off names of colleges she thought would be appropriate matches for me; places where I could play lacrosse as well as thrive academically—Bucknell,

Colgate, Connecticut College, Skidmore, Rutgers, Hobart and William Smith—rolled off her tongue and landed with a thud on the thinly carpeted floor of her office.

"How about Penn?" my father not so subtly suggested. "I think she could play for Penn and do the coursework. She can major in English and avoid the science and math classes."

That evening after dinner, my father called a friend of his who worked in Penn's alumni office and was active in the recruiting of alumni athletes. He assured my father he would follow up on my application and see it through. Soon, my high school lacrosse coaches contacted the head of women's lacrosse at Penn and put in a positive recommendation. I was promptly signed up for an SAT review course, and the nightly SAT workbook sessions began as religiously as dinner, which was served promptly every evening at 6:00. I felt pressure from my father to bring up my scores, but we never discussed the sudden need to learn how to take a standardized test in the first place, since the private school I attended barely gave grades. Like most things in my life growing up, I did the SAT review work because I was told to, because it was expected of me. There was little doubt in my mind of the payoff. Hard work, my father always said, paid off.

I applied to all of the schools on Helene Reynolds's list, and I remember visiting and interviewing at a few of them. At Rutgers, my father and I sat in a huge parking lot in a torrential downpour. Rutgers had an undergraduate program in education, and apparently, my father decided I was going to make a fine teacher. Law school seemed interesting to me, as did pediatric medicine. I don't think I had decided yet, but he had. I was dressed for my interview in blue wool knee-high socks, brown penny loafers that slipped off my narrow heels, a green-and-blue plaid wool skirt, and a white cotton button-down shirt uncomfortably tucked into the skirt. I was prepared, but I wasn't going into the admissions office.

"Dad, this is ridiculous," I told him. We sat next to each other, him in the driver's seat, his arm draped over the steering wheel, and me in the passenger seat, wishing I was anywhere but in that car, in that parking lot. Rain pelted against the hood and streamed in crooked rivulets down the windshield. "I'm not going to Rutgers. You know that. I don't even know why we're here. It's too big. I don't want to go to school in New Jersey."

My father took a deep breath and sighed like he had heard all this before because he had. "We're here, Jude. We have an appointment with someone in the admissions office in half an hour. You never know if you're going to like a school until you walk the campus. Let's just find the bookstore, grab an umbrella, and go to your interview." My father had warm brown eyes and thin black hair. He wore a white button-down shirt and khaki pants but no tie. His Penn hat, with the red-and-blue ribbon around the rim, was perched on his head. He spoke softly to me, never one to show frustration or anger, despite the fact he had driven three hours in the pouring rain. He didn't have to raise his voice. His disappointment in me was palpable. I could feel it rising off his skin like steam from a pot full of boiling water.

I stared out the passenger window at the large puddles forming on the black asphalt. I let my eyes scan the brick and concrete buildings that, to me, may as well have been office buildings or doctors' offices. I wasn't going to Rutgers. So I never got out of the car. My refusal felt like a tiny turn of a screw to the left in a much larger and more complicated control board that my father had made for me, which required me to always turn the screws to the right.

We didn't talk much on the ride home, but by the time we got there and my mother asked how it went, the story had been flattened and whitewashed into a mild comical tale about tromping around in the rain and how "we both knew she isn't going to Rutgers!"

What I had considered to be my small, successful rebellion became something my father had known about all along. It turns out it wasn't a rebellion at all.

MOVE-IN DAY AT PENN

1980

My room at Penn, a single joined by a bathroom to another single, was on the third floor of Cleeman Hall. "So lucky!" my mother swooned. "You have your own bathroom with Mindy!"

I guessed that was a good thing, although at the time, the only thing I thought was good about it was the possibility of locking myself in that bathroom and no one noticing my absence.

Against the odds, I had been accepted to Penn. For a while after the letter arrived, I was proud and excited. It was a big deal in my senior class at the Park School in Baltimore to have been admitted to Penn. And not only that, but I was also a freshman recruit on the field hockey and lacrosse teams. But now that we were standing in my dorm room, I felt like a complete imposter. Who was I fooling? The admissions office had made a mistake; these people were going to see right through me.

My mother helped me unroll a cushy blue carpet while my father went down the hall and arranged for me to have a phone in my room—unusual for back then, when the hall phone was the norm. Then my mother made my bed, and I hung a few pictures on the wall of friends and family, along with a large Marimekko fabric-covered, bright green mural, something with panels about the weather. When I think back on that wall hanging, it should have been a sign to my parents and me that I was not ready for this move. I took my shampoo, toothpaste, and towels into the bathroom, making sure to leave plenty of room for Mindy, who, it turns out, was from Erie, Pennsylvania, and had arrived by herself with only a suitcase of clothes and was already off mingling with our neighbors in Cleeman Hall.

"Well," my father said, his blue button-down shirt showing perspiration marks under the armpits. It was Philadelphia in late August, after all. "I think this is it. Why don't you turn on your radio and listen to some music, or maybe go find Denise? Isn't she moving into the dorm across the quad?" Denise was a friend from my high school who was also a freshman at Penn.

"That's a good idea!" my mother said with a little too much enthusiasm. "Why don't you go visit Denise? The two of you can figure some things out together." With those words, she stood up from the extra-long twin-size bed, wrapped her arms around me, gave me a squeeze, and said, "You're going to be just fine."

I could not speak or I would break into tears, so I nodded and motioned for my parents to leave. I couldn't watch them, but I heard their footsteps as they walked out the large wooden door of my sweltering room, down three flights of narrow steps, and out the arched doorway. As soon as they left, I felt an odd sense of relief. I could do whatever I wanted to do—go see Denise, cry in the bathroom, wander around the city of Philadelphia. But I couldn't shake the feeling that I wasn't going to make it here, that

I should have always been doing something else at college, something other than what it was I was doing. Because whatever I did, it wasn't enough.

Now I wonder, years later: Was my own son sitting on his bed, on his first day in his college dorm, thinking the exact same thing?

The stain was proving difficult to wash out.

COLLEGE FOR JAMES

2010

James may have been trying to flip the switch to Off, but I was still on Go. Like my father before me, I wasn't going to let a few points on James's test scores get in the way of his chances of being accepted into "the best" college he could go to, even if "the best" colleges in the nation weren't necessarily the best colleges for James. I was determined to control him in the same way my father controlled me. I instructed James to fill out the form for the Williams College recruiting camp and to stay in touch with the coach. Meanwhile, I made plane reservations to fly into the Rutland Vermont Airport and rented a car. Not just any car—I rented a canary yellow Pontiac Firebird. If James didn't want to go to Williams, at least he would enjoy the ride.

When James and I visited the campus, there was one main street in walking distance from the manicured quads of the college. We passed a barber shop, a few small restaurants, the Williams College Bookstore, and a coffee shop. "Is that it?" James asked me when we came to the end of the street, which dead-ended at a narrow river. "No way am I going here. There's nothing to do."

"Give it a chance, James. I'm sure the kids find their own fun on campus. It's beautiful!" I felt frustrated that James failed to see the beauty in this serene college town. I was disappointed that he didn't even want to put in the effort to get into a school like Williams.

If he really didn't want to go, he might not try his hardest on the soccer field the next day. And if the coaches didn't want him as a recruit, he wasn't getting into Williams. I heard my father's voice in my ear: *Here's his chance to go to a top-tier school, Jude. Use the soccer to get him in. Once he's in, he'll be fine. He'll love it, just like you did at Penn.*

It didn't occur to me that it took me years to feel like I fit in at Penn, and by then, some damage had been done to my confidence and my self-esteem. It was a thoroughly exhausting experience. But I was still chanting, "Keep a-goin'."

The next morning, while I wandered around the art museum, James played in front of the Williams' soccer staff, who never followed up with him. He didn't go to Williams. But I remained determined, in the same way I suppose my father had stayed the path, that James would get into a "good" school and play soccer in college. I performed this whole routine one more time at Brown University when James was invited to attend their soccer camp the summer before his senior year of high school. What I know now about being "invited" to a recruiting camp is that, often, it has more to do with making money for the soccer program than it has to do with recruiting players to the team. "What the hell am I doing here, Mom?" he said to me from a hall pay phone at Brown.

"Ummm, I think you are playing soccer in front of the Brown coaches to see if you might be a soccer recruit for them?"

"Nope, Mom. Not at all. There are guys here from Argentina and a ton of kids from California. They are basically professional soccer players, Mom. There is no way I am getting recruited to play for Brown. They have guys here from all over the world. What don't you understand about that? Why did you make me come to this? It's hot as shit in the dorms, I don't have a fan, and there is no point to this."

I heard the voice of my father drowning out any rational thoughts I might have had about James's chances of playing soccer for Brown. *To allow him to come home is to admit defeat. Quitting is not an option. You never know, Jude—if he plays well enough tomorrow, one of the Brown coaches just might help him get in.*

If you don't learn from history, it has a way of repeating itself.

MOVE-IN DAY: COLORADO COLLEGE

AUGUST 2010

The whole family—Daniel, James, Julia, Nathan, and I—flew to Colorado College in Colorado Springs to drop James off. Because we couldn't fit all five of us in one hotel room, we reserved a separate room for James the night before we moved him into his dorm. The whole flight to Colorado and that afternoon, he seemed nervous, his words clipped and short, his temper near the edge. But these were signs only we, his parents, sensed. On the outside, it appeared he couldn't wait to be independent, free from our curfews, consequences, and counselors.

As soon as we checked into the hotel in the late afternoon, James wanted to go find one of his teammates from California—by himself. When we had dinner with a few of his fellow soccer recruits, James was smooth as the butter he smeared on his rolls. He flipped his bangs out of his face, snickered at his younger brother and sister's attempts to talk to his friends. He couldn't even wait twenty-four hours to get high in his dorm room.

From our own hotel room, Daniel and I thought we smelled smoke. I tapped on the door to James's adjoining room, turned the knob, and pushed the door open. There he sat, joint between his thumb and pointer finger, at the shiny wooden desk, the one with the King James Bible tucked into the top drawer.

Clueless. Entitled. Doomed. These were some of the words that ran through my head about James at that moment. It was like he was picking at the scar until it bled.

"It's no big deal, Mom. We're in Colorado. It's practically legal." He placed the joint on the glass ashtray in front of him, his eyes bloodshot and half closed. He leaned back on two legs of the desk chair, his feet resting on the edge of the desk. He might have fallen over backward but for the way the legs of the chair dug into the carpeting. His whole demeanor was relaxed, as if his body was shouting to me, "Chill out."

"What the hell, James?" I spat out at him, my voice an angry whisper. "Your brother and sister are in the next room. It's not legal, and you are in a hotel!"

James tilted his head and looked back at me, as if changing his perspective might calm me down.

I wasn't going to miss this routine.

I picked up the joint from the ashtray, walked it over to the toilet, dropped it in the water, and flushed it. The room was dim. He had not opened the curtains, but I saw him shake his head slowly and step toward his bed.

"We're leaving for dinner in an hour," I said, "see if you can get yourself showered, cleaned up, and ready to go. Maybe even pretend you want to be with us." I walked out of his room and shut the door behind me.

This did not bode well for the next four years at Colorado College. I had visions of him realizing he wanted to play soccer more than he wanted to smoke weed, that he would find a professor and a class that would motivate him and come to ignite his interest in French, or Buddhist studies, or really anything. But those were *my* dreams for him, not his. And they were about to be blown away in the whirl of the sweet smoke of a joint.

The next day, the coaches welcomed the new players to the Colorado College soccer "family." The director of athletics informed us of some highlights about the upcoming season and what the coaches expected of players in the two weeks of preseason. It would be hot and grueling, the head coach warned. "But your boys will make it through. They will forge lifelong friendships on this team and learn lessons not taught in any classrooms. We are honored to have each and every one of your sons. This is a great group of young men, and we can't wait to get on the field and work with them."

When I hugged James goodbye in that field house, I wept.

But what James didn't know was that my tears were not ones of joy and excitement for him; I wept because I was afraid. So afraid that he would fail.

NOT A GOOD BET

DECEMBER 2009

"There is a 30 percent chance this will be the best thing that ever happened to him," Daniel said to me after the official acceptance letter from Colorado College had arrived in the mail. "There is a 50 percent chance he will make it through. And there is a 20 percent chance this will be an unmitigated disaster."

We thought that because Colorado College used the block system for classes, where students take one course at a time for three weeks, it might be a good match for James's ability to focus his attention for short bursts. We thought that the structure of his day at CC—classes in the morning and practice all afternoon—would keep James busy and tired enough to put an end to his marijuana obsession. We thought that making new friends on the soccer team, maybe joining an outdoor club, snowboarding, mountain biking, would lead him down a new and different path.

We thought wrong.

IS THIS HOW WE GOT HERE?

NOVEMBER 1991

Family lore says that when James was a baby, I dropped him on his head. But that's not true. When he was less than a year old, he was crying in his crib, drenched in sweat, zipped up in red terry cloth pajamas. In my half sleep, I took him from the crib, changed his diaper, and held him close to me, my mind already in the kitchen pouring the Enfamil formula into a bottle and warming it up in the microwave oven.

I walked down the steps, one hand under James's bottom, one hand cradling his head, pulling him next to my chest. I liked the smell of the top of his baby head. When I realized I was sliding down the stairs instead of stepping down them, I held James tightly and made sure he didn't fall off of me. We landed at the bottom near the front door. My left foot throbbed, and my big toe stuck out in an unnatural position. James screamed, but he was perched in the exact same position in my arms that he'd started in. He never hit his head.

There was a time James did hit his head, but he managed that all by himself. At his six-month baby visit, James lay on his back on a green, padded examination table while I waited for Dr. Donner. I stood next to James, staring at pictures of balloons and framed medical degrees. I am sure I had one hand on James's body, but maybe not, because somehow, he rolled over.

Although I did not see him fall, I heard him hit the linoleum tile floor. There was a thud and a sudden, piercing scream that echoed off the walls. I was alone and terrified. What kind of mother allows her baby to tumble off the exam table at the pediatrician's? I was sure I was about to be reported to social services. I pressed James as close to my body as I could and bounced him gently and whispered, "Shhh, shhh, you're okay," into his ear.

James's screams finally brought Dr. Donner into the room for the not-so-well-anymore baby visit. James had a small bump on his forehead that quickly turned from red to pale blue. Dr. Donner shined a tiny light into James's eyes and moved it up and down, right and left. Then he pressed James's head and announced he would be fine. James's screams subsided into tiny hiccups, and splotchy red patches covered his face. His eyes leaked tears for the rest of the exam. No concussion protocols existed then.

A nurse gave James his vaccines, and I answered Dr. Donner's questions about James's eating habits (constant and demanding), his mobility (crawling like a wind-up toy), and his sleep patterns (is not sleeping a pattern?)

That was it. Take him home and keep an eye on his head. Call the office if I noticed anything out of the ordinary.

It would be many years before I chose to notice anything out of the ordinary about James. And by then, Dr. Donner had retired.

NATURE QUEST WILDERNESS THERAPY

SOMEWHERE IN SOUTHERN UTAH, FEBRUARY 2012

I feel that marijuana has only recently become a major obstacle for me in terms of being productive in the college setting. It also has had financial implications due to my misdemeanor and arrest and my extensive interest in spending money on glass and new exciting things that are being made in the marijuana industry. My parents believe this is true and that it is preventing me from reaching my potential as well as causing more anxiety in my life and my family's life. They think that weed has made me someone who cannot be trusted and is simply living the life of an addict. I seriously believe it is my own decision to use that has led to my recent failure in college as opposed to pot being readily available or the environment being a "bad" one. I have wasted my parents' money by not fully applying myself at one of the most expensive colleges in the country. Weed use has made me spend my parents' money that I have not earned on paraphernalia, pot, and weed-related items/clothing. In the long run, I feel it may have somewhat of an impact on my life which I am willing to accept. My parents believe it will prevent me from achieving anything to be proud of in the future.

TWO WEEKS

SEPTEMBER 2010

That's all it took.

"Mom?"

"Hey, bud!" I was surprised to hear from James because I knew he had just arrived back at campus after a week-long camping trip with his soccer team. They'd started preseason practices the day after.

"How's it going?" I asked with the same hopeful enthusiasm in my voice that I remember my own parents had on the phone with me when I was in college.

It was as if my optimism might deflect any unfortunate news he may have to tell me. As if maybe, when he heard the sound of my voice, he would change his mind about whatever it was he was going to say.

"Well, not so good." He sounded down but not as bad as he should have sounded based on what he was about to tell me.

"What's wrong, James? Are you okay?"

"I mean, I'm okay. But I'm kinda in the hospital at Colorado Springs. I'm here getting fluids and stuff. I think I was dehydrated, and I kept throwing up and I couldn't stop, so I went to the health clinic at CC, and they told me to go to the emergency room at the hospital here, so that's where I am."

"Did you get sick on the camping trip?" I sensed there was more to this story. I felt like James had just kicked over the first domino. I wasn't panicked or shocked; it was more like grave disappointment.

"Yeah, I mean, I started throwing up on the camping trip, and the coaches told me to keep drinking water, that it was altitude. But then, even after we got back, I couldn't practice because I was, like, so weak. So I missed most of preseason."

"Did you talk to the coach? Is he letting you try out even though preseason is over?"

James was calling me from an emergency room from a hospital in Colorado Springs, explaining to me that he was dehydrated enough to be admitted to a hospital, but I couldn't wrap my head around the idea that he may not be playing soccer for Colorado College.

He would recover from the dehydration; that was an easy fix, and it would only take a few more hours. But being cut from the team? That could have some long-term consequences. It felt to me like the bottom block had been yanked from the tower. It was shaky but still standing. Everything that might keep James thriving at Colorado College just got kicked to the side of the road. There would be no structure to his day without soccer practice, his friends would no longer be the members of the team, and it would be easy for him to fall back into a daily marijuana habit. Soccer was the glue holding this project together.

"I mean, basically, I didn't make the team because I wasn't there for most of the tryout. It's fine, Mom. I can play club soccer if I want. Or maybe I'll just chill out and not play for this year. It's fine."

"Are you okay? Do you need Dad or me to fly out and help you?"

His calm acceptance was suspicious to me. Twelve years of soccer, and the promise of a college soccer career blown in a week, and he was "fine" with it? I shook my head even though James couldn't see me. I didn't understand why he wasn't more disappointed, frustrated, and determined to try to play again, maybe because I was feeling all of those emotions for him. Or maybe I was just feeling all of those emotions for me.

"No, Mom, please. They told me I would be out of here in a few hours. I feel much better already. I think I was just really dehydrated. You know, like I didn't drink enough water on the campout for the first few days of practice. I'll be fine. I'll call you later."

"Okay, bud. It's just that I'm worried about how you will spend your free time now. I mean, as a recruit, he wanted you on the team just a few weeks ago. Is there anyone else in your class who didn't make the team?"

You would have thought I was the one getting cut from this soccer team. I was indignant.

"Yeah, that kid Andrew from California. I don't know. The coach just told me that he didn't get to see me play enough during preseason because I got sick, and he hopes I'll try out again next year. I'll be fine, Mom. I'll talk to you later."

Maybe I would call Andrew's mother and find out what he was going to do now with wide-open afternoons and hours of free time. No, who was I kidding? James was in college, and I was not calling anyone's mother. I sat down at our kitchen table and, from the tips of my fingers right down to the hollow feeling in my stomach, I knew this news was going to topple the shaky tower that was James.

I WON'T TURN ON THE LIGHTS

To call me an accomplice or an enabler to James's substance use disorder would not be inaccurate. Although something felt off when he told me things like, "I think I was dehydrated," I wanted to believe him. It was possible, I reassured myself. I might have also believed that pigs could fly if, at the time, he had told me that was true.

To accept what was reported to me by him, I had to deny a few things I knew were true. A healthy nineteen-year-old boy in excellent physical shape does not wind up dehydrated in a hospital. A boy who routinely traveled to Utah every winter since he was seven years old to ski mountains at ten thousand feet with no symptoms of altitude sickness does not land in a hospital with altitude sickness in need of fluids. A recruited soccer player, a kid who earned one of ten slots on the coach's list for admissions, doesn't suddenly not make the team. The stage was set at Colorado College. But from where I sat in Baltimore, the house lights were off.

I would never be able to see through the darkness if I didn't allow my eyes to adjust to the light. But it takes effort, and sometimes even pain, to do that, and I wanted to continue to move around in the dark, so I did. I believed what James told us.

Because I am sitting now in a place where the house lights are on, I can see the stage, and I believe the reason James suffered from dehydration and nausea two weeks into his freshman year was due to marijuana withdrawal. When James was in high school and we'd travel to Utah to ski, he predictably would throw up on the drive from the airport to our ski house. Frequently, when we went out to dinner, and sometimes at the house in the morning before we left for the mountain, he would throw up. If James could land some pot in Utah, from a ski instructor or a friend of a friend, the vomiting would stop. But since he could not bring the weed with him on the airplane, he threw up until he could find some pot. At the time, we too called it altitude sickness.

James knew he would be drug tested when he tried out for the soccer team at Colorado College, and he knew he would be randomly tested throughout the season. I give him credit for trying. If his last joint was the one he enjoyed in that hotel room adjoining mine, he was probably experiencing withdrawal symptoms within the week, which can include anxiety, headaches, vomiting, depression, and stomach pain. According to Peter Grinspoon, MD, at Harvard Health, proponents of cannabis often dismiss the possibility of withdrawal syndrome. One psychiatrist I spoke to in Colorado Springs explained to us that James could not possibly be physically addicted to marijuana because it is not an addictive drug. I do not believe this for one second. Either way, when James called me from that hospital, he didn't want to stop smoking weed, and he had no intention of trying.

STOP THIS TRAIN, I WANT TO GET OFF

OCTOBER 2011

It's not like we didn't see it coming. But the finality of it still came as a shock. It was early October of James's sophomore year at Colorado College when we got the call. "Hey, Mom," he said, "I need to tell you something. Can you put Dad on the phone? I'm not okay. I want to come home. I'm messed up. I can't do this. I need help."

I sat down at our family room table in Baltimore and motioned with my head for Daniel, who was sitting across from me, to take the phone. I am sure there was silence on the phone, but I remember a strange sense of relief, a tingling, like what honesty would feel like if you could touch it.

In that silence was a letting go, warm and sweet like the smell of bread baking. The relief was palpable. If we had been unable to connect the dots until now, the image became clear to us at that moment. Suddenly, it all made sense. James couldn't stop using by himself, and he was calling to ask for help.

"James, you are doing the right thing," Daniel said. "I'm going to come get you, okay? Stay where you are. Are you safe right now? Do you need help this minute?"

"No, no, I'm okay. I just need to come home." James was sloppy-crying and sniffling and hiccupping. "I don't want to do this anymore."

"Okay, bud. I'm making a reservation. Is someone there with you right now?"

"Yeah, yeah. My roommate's here."

"Okay, good. We'll figure it out when I get there," Daniel told him. He handed the phone back to me.

"Bud, don't hang up," I said. "I want you to call me if you need to, okay? I'll be right here for you. Please call if you want to talk while you wait for Dad to get there, okay?"

Daniel was already on his laptop, checking for flights to Colorado Springs.

"Okay," James said. "I will. Please let me come home. I can't do this anymore."

I hung up the phone, and at that moment, I thought how brave James was to yank himself off the track. I surprised myself by feeling nothing but relief and empathy for him. My usual reaction might have been disappointment or frustration or embarrassment for both of us, but this felt more like a birth, like something had been released and something else had taken its place. Something that we had been waiting a long time for.

Let's call it honesty.

ONLY LOVE CAN BREAK YOUR HEART

As his mother, I believed it was my job to save James. I would do whatever it took to help him get sober and learn to live a healthy, productive life. What I did not fully comprehend was that I couldn't force James to stop using drugs and alcohol. No amount of money, love, persuasion, pleading, begging, fighting, bargaining, praying, or wishing on my part could lead James down the path to sobriety. No one and nothing could convince me at the time that only James could help James.

WE HAVE LOST CONTROL

DECEMBER 2012

James took a leave of absence from Colorado College and moved home. Daniel and I consulted a trusted psychologist and had hopes that after some outpatient addiction therapy, a schedule involving a job, and boundaries around where James went and when, he would be able to return to Colorado College for the spring semester. It turns out it takes more than a few rules and a little hope to keep an addict from using.

It was about 10:30 at night during the first week that James was home. Daniel and I stood in the dining room, mail scattered across the polished wooden dining table because that is where we tossed the mail until we read it. James had been in his room doing something at his computer when I heard him jog down the front stairs, taking some two at a time. When he saw Daniel and me in the dining room, his hand was already on the handle of the front door.

He tossed his head to the right to clear the hair out of his eyes. "I'm goin' to Lerner's," he said. Max Lerner was a friend from high school who lived about two miles from us and was home from St. Mary's College in Maryland for winter break.

James knew he was not allowed to leave the house after 10:00 p.m., and in a calmer moment, he had agreed to follow that rule. Daniel shouted after him that he was not going out and that he needed to get back inside the house "NOW."

"The fuck I am!" James screamed back at both of us, slamming the front door behind him.

I flinched. The sound of the door was like a gunshot a few feet from where I was standing. I quickly thought about where Julia and Nathan were. Nathan was sleeping over at a friend's house, and Julia was due home from a movie by 11:30. Not that they hadn't heard battles like this before between James and us, but why make them listen to one more?

I heard the engine turn over and the car drive out of the driveway. "I'm going to hide the knives," Daniel said. "Who knows what he'll do? It's either that or change the locks."

I shook my head in disbelief. How did we get here? James was taller than Daniel, certainly stronger than I was, and determined to get what he wanted. My heart raced, and my eyes darted around the room, spotting objects that previously looked benign to me but now turned into weapons. I knew if we'd ever had control over James, we had surely lost it now.

I'M GLAD YOU ASKED

"Did you realize you had an addict on your hands?
Were you ready to get honest with yourself?"

I could say, at this point, that honesty and hope were tied up in a knot. I could say, when it's your child, determination and hope look a lot like denial. I could say I still had plans for James to graduate from Colorado College, to stay in peak physical condition, to have a career, to love a partner, to have children. I could say, If this were your child, would you give up on those dreams? I knew James was an addict. I wanted to say, Don't confuse blind faith for blindness.

"Did you realize you had an addict on your hands?
Were you ready to get honest with yourself?"

I did. I will never give up on this kid, but I had to learn to make boundaries.

NATURE QUEST WILDERNESS THERAPY

SOMEWHERE IN SOUTHERN UTAH, JANUARY 9, 2012

I am here at Nature Quest because I either had to live on my own with nowhere to go or get myself together and gain my parents' trust back. My parents and I met with a therapist to decide what "Rehab program" would be best for me. My parents see pot as holding me back and preventing me from reaching my potential. They firmly want me to stop using for a while and believe I can't stop. I am here to show them I can stop and that I just need to regain focus and not use it as an outlet for my problems. I need to find other ways to deal with things that bother me or cause problems for me. I wasn't resistant to coming to Nature Quest but I also am not interested in going to a rehab program. I've always felt in control and overpowered through conflicts or found ways around my problems, not always for the better, however.

ULTIMATUM, THE FIRST ONE

JANUARY 2012

Sending a child to wilderness therapy wasn't a chapter in *What to Expect When You're Expecting*. My own mother never warned me that, one day, I would have to tell my son he couldn't live with us anymore. I never asked my friends over coffee for advice on how to kick my kid out of the house. It wasn't a topic that bubbled up, like whether to use day care, or how to start potty training, or later, how to rent a tuxedo for the prom.

Within a few weeks of returning home from college, James had been fired from waiting tables at Donna's Café, a local restaurant in Baltimore, and had concluded that landscaping was hard work. He had been arrested for possession of marijuana at a skateboard park in Utah. His outbursts were unpredictable and frightening, and he refused to go to treatment. He kept his own hours, which meant he was up all night and asleep until early afternoon. The boundaries we attempted to enforce meant nothing to him. I didn't know how to help him.

I understood that my son had substance use disorder, and I was willing to do whatever I had to do to help him beat this disease. It did not occur to me that my son had mental illness. It did not occur to me to look behind the behavior or beyond the drugs for a cause of the drug use, beyond the fact that the substances were addictive and he was an addict. No doctor or therapist ever mentioned to me the term "dual diagnosis." Call me naive, blind, or dumb, but I was only focused on drug rehabilitation.

Because I was scared and felt alone, I sought advice from psychologists, addiction counselors, and educational consultants.

"Throw him out," trusted psychologists told me.

"You're being used," addiction counselors warned. "You didn't cause this, and you can't cure him. He's not going to stop using until he hits rock bottom. You're fueling his habit. Tell him he either gets help and follows the rules or you're kicking him out of the house."

Asking James to leave the house remains the most difficult thing I have ever said to any of my children. In hindsight, it was the best decision Daniel and I have made. In many ways, we were lucky. In the end, he chose to get help. And we could afford to send him. He was not enthusiastic about going to Nature Quest, but he did get on the plane with nothing but a backpack slung over his shoulder and, I later learned, a tiny piece of paper tucked into his back pocket with the phone number of a friend who might pick him up in Salt Lake City.

Just in case.

GOOD LUCK TO YOU

JANUARY 2012

After dropping James off at Baltimore/Washington International Airport, I felt the need to know that someone from Nature Quest was going to be at the other end of the flight. I wanted reassurance they had him, that he was in their hands. "So you'll meet him at the Salt Lake Airport, right? Someone will be there?" I opened the door to our house in Baltimore and looked up at the sky, holding the phone between my ear and shoulder.

"We'll be there." The director of the program was trying to reassure me from his home base in St. George, Utah, roughly two hours from Salt Lake City. "And we will do everything in our power to get him to come with us. James is twenty years old, so he has the right to walk away. But look, he got on the plane, and he agreed to try it."

"Okay, true," I sighed into the phone. "But call me when you have him, please."

I would be lying if I said I was heartbroken to have James out of the house. I remember feeling a sense of relief, a calm wave filling my body after he left. As long as he was in the woods of southern Utah, he was not storming around in my house, slamming doors, arguing, or asking for money. I would no longer be lying awake at night wondering where he was and if he would make it home alive. No more attempts to place boundaries between a dog and his bone. Julia and Nathan deserved to live in a peaceful home, and they were about to receive that gift.

After I'd hung up with the director of Nature Quest, I went back inside and sank into the sofa in the family room. If you have not experienced living with an addict while trying to maintain some semblance of family life or even just keeping up with your own life, sending a child away for someone else to deal with might seem irresponsible or neglectful. It might have appeared as if we were passing James's problems off to someone else. But from where I am now, many years later, I still view this decision to send him to Utah as the kindest thing I have ever done for myself, for my family, and for James.

"Good luck to you," I uttered to no one in our family room. I meant it both for James and for every counselor in that program.

NATURE QUEST WILDERNESS THERAPY

SOMEWHERE IN SOUTHERN UTAH, JANUARY 10, 2012

Today is my second day out in the wilderness. I didn't realize how frozen and cold everything would get overnight. Being alone with myself and unable to communicate with the group has been painfully boring and making time go by extra slow. I hope I move on past earth phase relatively soon. Throughout today I hope to have a good meeting with my therapist. Having a mentor has been helpful in terms of having something to look forward to and getting back to the real world. Last night was pretty bright because of the full moon, hopefully, more stars will be visible tonight and in the upcoming nights. Hoping today is the last day of earth phase.

CALL FROM A SATELLITE PHONE

JANUARY 2012

Because James's group was hunkered down in the woods of Utah, miles away from any town, our contact with him was limited to letter writing. Once a week, however, we spoke with his therapist, who saw James at least twice a week in his office under a tree on a log. After two weeks, James was allowed to call us once, using a satellite phone provided by one of his counselors. The day and time of the call were predetermined. It was only allowed once in the twelve weeks James was in the program.

"Mom?"

"Hey, James! It's great to hear your voice. How are you doing?" Daniel and I had set up a landline phone between us and placed it on speaker. We didn't want to risk bad reception on a cell phone, and we wanted to be together when we spoke to him. As soon as I heard James's voice, an old enthusiasm and perkiness set into my body. The last few weeks had allowed me to reclaim the routine structure of my life and, far from feeling guilty for sending him away, I was optimistic that James would emerge from this program cured and ready to return to college.

He sounded very far away because he was.

"How do you think I'm doing? You and Dad sent me to *Holes*. I hike all day, and then I have to make a fire in the forest without matches. Ever tried that? It's freezing cold, and we don't even sleep in tents."

I wanted to say, That's why it's called wilderness therapy. And that Daniel and I had bought into it fully with our hearts and our pocketbooks. Instead, I said, "*Holes*? What are you talking about?"

"*Holes*. Remember the book I read about that prison camp for boys, where all they do is dig *holes* all day and try not to get bit by scorpions? Well, that's what you sent me to. I hope you're happy."

I could hear the anger in his voice loud and clear, but I had to laugh. He had always loved that book. I remembered how I dumped on my parents when I went to summer camp. I wanted them to feel guilty about sending me away, to know they had made a terrible mistake. I knew at some level this was James's plan too. Nature Quest was no five-star hotel, but Daniel and I had thoroughly researched it. We'd spoken at length to the director, the therapist, and the program coordinator. We believed in the entire philosophy behind wilderness therapy, and we were convinced James was a good candidate. He had always been a visceral kid; he learned by moving and doing. He loved the outdoors, had always been happiest when he was mountain biking, skiing, hiking. I couldn't imagine him trying to recover in an inpatient hospital, attending meetings in an air-conditioned conference room, sleeping in a small bedroom. I didn't feel sorry for James as I listened to him on the satellite phone. Not one bit.

"I remember that book, bud. It's funny you think Nature Quest is like *Holes*. What are your days like? Tell me something good." I wanted to keep James on the phone, but I wasn't going to listen to him complain about the program. There was no other option here, and I desperately wanted to hear him sound like he was making an effort to adapt, trying to cooperate with his counselors, doing some introspective work.

"I don't know. I guess it's nice to sleep under the stars. The people are pretty cool. Did you talk to my therapist, Pete? I like him." There it was: a spark that just needed to be fanned. My old conviction that this kid could get back on a track, any track at this point, kicked in, and I believed he could do it.

"We are speaking to him this week. Settle in, bud. There's a lot to learn. We have faith in you and in the program. Stick with that fire lighting. You'll get it."

"Yeah, we have to bust a flame using a rock and a string. It's really hard." His voice got softer like it did before he cried. It was okay if he cried. He should cry for God's sake. What he was doing was very difficult work, and it was about time he came to grips with the fact that this wasn't going to be comfortable. He had dug himself a deep hole, and maybe he was realizing it wasn't going to be so easy to find his way out.

"You always do what you set out to do. Keep writing us letters, and we'll write back, okay?" There it was again, in me: "Keep a-goin'" James. Even if it's writing letters and busting fires, do it well. I understood this was not writing papers and playing soccer in college, but to me, even these actions for James were a means to an end. If he thrived at Nature Quest, did what he was supposed to do, grew in the ways he needed to grow, this would be a temporary detour. He could return to college, be a normal kid.

Reader, still no one mentioned the words "anxiety," "depression," "ADHD," or "bipolar disorder" to us in the same breath as they did "substance use disorder." Do I wonder now how I missed the signs? Sometimes, but I will never know if James's drug use was the result of self-medicating for bipolar disorder, or if the mental illness triggered his drug use. And there is no use in trying to determine if it was the chicken or the egg. No one knows the answer to that riddle. That's why it's a good one.

"Okay, I will. I miss you guys. Tell Julia and Nathan I said hi. When are you coming to visit?"

We were allowed to visit after he'd been at the program for eight weeks. At that point, he would either be allowed to graduate from Nature Quest or he would stay another month.

"Let's see how it goes. Don't think about weeks from now, James. Focus on why you are there, and deal with what you are doing day by day. We'll write you soon, okay? We love you very much." I felt proud of him, happy for him, and hopeful. Maybe I was trying to tie the bow too tightly, but I felt like we were at least stepping up on the ladder and not falling off.

"Love you too, Mom. Love you, Dad. Bye."

Daniel and I hung up, looked at each other, and smiled. The call was funny, not too far from what we expected, and his voice sounded strong and even. Hearing his voice, I missed him. But I missed the James I used to know, not the one we sent to wilderness therapy. I felt relieved he was hundreds of miles away without a drink or a joint in two weeks, like a door that has been cracked open just enough to see a slice of light. I even thought I had heard a little of the old James bubble up in our conversation.

I was still very willing to believe I had control over James's recovery.

NATURE QUEST WILDERNESS THERAPY

SOMEWHERE IN SOUTHERN UTAH, FEBRUARY 2012

I am here because I am an entitled MOFO.

LETTER HOME FROM JAMES

NATURE QUEST WILDERNESS THERAPY,
JANUARY 19, 2012

Dear Mom and Dad,

First I would like to start off by reflecting upon Dad's letter because it is the one I chose to read first. Unexpectedly, it was more forgiving just because Mom is more exhausted and closer to the point of completely giving up out of losing her patience, which is valid at this point in our relationship.

I fully understand why you sent me to Nature Quest and why it may have been difficult for both of you. Most of the kids and parents I have encountered here have expressed the same inability to cope with their child's actions and need to step back because they feel like they are only furthering the problem. It was not a surprise to me that you listed and described my recent and past events that reveal my rage, loss of motivation, lack of responsible spending, secrecy, academic failure, and lastly, legal trouble. I recognize how my rage impacts the family's emotional safety and disrupts the sense of peace that a family should provide for its members. I was well aware that neither you nor mom would try and stop me while I was home because of the possibility of a physical altercation. My secrecy, stealing, and excessive partying that you mentioned are spot on and truly describe my actions while at Colorado College and over the summer. You are absolutely correct about the savings account; however, the storage unit was used for legitimate purposes. After being sober here at Nature Quest, and identifying why I chose to use, I am on the same page that I enjoyed the mood-altering effects of the drugs I have done. I also realize how stupid it is to use tobacco, especially considering the state that Grampsy is in right now.

As soon as you mentioned the pictures, I began to break down crying. I couldn't help but think I reached my prime during my senior year of high school and I have been on a slow and steady decline ever since.

When thinking and reflecting on the overall decline of my lifestyle, physical traits, and personality I have come to realize how I have been setting myself up for failure and my family for exhaustion and disappointment. This part of your letter, Dad, made me sink down into the ultimate lows I experience when expressing my sense of failure and the distrust that exists between us because of how I have acted and impacted everyone around me, including myself.

Mom, when I describe my relationship with my parents to staff and fellow clients here at Nature Quest, I have been informing everyone that you are the one who I ask if I can do things because you tend to be more lenient and fickle than Dad. You hit the nail on the head when expressing how you normally feel and act toward me. Your recent shift to a fed-up and angry and tired mother is understandable after reading Dad's letter as well as the physical and emotional destruction I have caused to you, Dad, Julia, and Nathan. The choice words I screamed out of pure rage and anger have no actual meaning or relation to you or anyone. I merely was out of control and frustrated with my new restraints after being arrested. Also, the step you and Dad took when you decided that I needed to be sent away frustrated me beyond belief and made me completely disregard how my actions and choices would affect the family and those around me because I knew I was going away, and it was past the point of no return. How I have impacted Nathan is something that I am shameful of and want to write to him about. I am working on writing him an apology letter, but it is very emotionally challenging for me to accept what harm I have caused him. I am relieved to hear that Julia is made of steel and has been able to persevere through my destructive and inappropriate behavior. I love Nathan and Julia dearly and want to mend how I negatively impacted them. I want to be closer to both of them and be viewed in a positive light from their perception.

I am happy to learn how to be joyous and manage my stress without illicit substances. My sober time here, (only 11 days) has helped me reconnect with my emotions and draw connections between my drug abuse and its role in my life. The way I have looked at my drug use in the past has been clouded by a lot of THC and twisted thinking. I never came to you and Dad for help because of my denial that I had a problem and my love for my new useless hobby, weed and hash oil. Your perception of me this past summer was spot on. I was near the pit of my downward spiral caused by drugs and my ignorance to admit I was wrong.

You are right about ending our arguments about marijuana. It has brought me down and got me nowhere valuable. I realize my potential and that you still love me and always will. My personality and sharp sense of humor have been dulled by the drugs and exhausted you physically and mentally. You were right to send me here to rediscover my true self and accept, not push away, the love you guys (my family) offer me.

Love,
James

YOU CAN'T TELL BY LOOKING

James and Family,

This book is a small token to remind you of all that you've accomplished at Nature Quest. We hope the memories of your wilderness experience will last a lifetime. We are grateful for having been a part of your journey and wish you all the best.

The Nature Quest Team

I am flipping through the small book of photographs we were gifted when James left Nature Quest. I have held on to it for eleven years now; two of the pages are loose and fall out if I hold the book the wrong way. I keep it on my desk, this thin book, between the journals and notebooks he kept while he was there.

You can't tell from looking at these snapshots that Daniel and I flew out to Utah as soon as the directors gave us the word that it was okay to visit him, which was about eight weeks into the program. You can't tell that when we arrived at the program's headquarters, a small cabin near the river in St. George, we were handed a tin cup, a headlamp, a sleeping bag, down booties, and a tarp. You can't tell from looking that the zipper on my sleeping bag was broken, and all night, my feet kicked the bag open, and I gave up, pulled out my Jodi Picoult book, turned my head lamp on, and read. You can't tell how hard I hugged James when we arrived at the site and he smelled like smoke. You can't tell from the pictures how happy I was to see him in the morning, dressed in a bright orange sherpa coat, a navy blue wool cap, and thin khaki pants. You can't tell how badly I wanted him to be better, and how desperately I wanted him to come home with us. You can't tell how proud I was of him when he taught me how to bust a fire with no matches, only a string attached to a bent piece of wood, and a rock. You can't tell from looking how shocked and sad I was when we sat down with James and his therapist told us that James was not ready to be released from the program yet, and furthermore, when he was ready to go, he could not go back to Colorado College; he would need to go to a halfway house. You can't tell from looking that Mike was serious about this advice, that the first twenty-four hours after James left Nature Quest would be the highest risk for him to relapse. You can't tell from looking how overwhelmed I felt with this information and how many questions I had running through my mind: Where would James go after Nature Quest if not back to school? Where would he go between Nature Quest and any halfway house we might find? What was a halfway house, anyway? You can't tell from looking how slowly my heart sank and with what drag, how deep the hole in my gut, and how heavy I felt as we walked away from the private meeting, which was on a log in a clearing under a tree. You can't tell from looking at any pictures how relieved I was to return my supplies to the sturdy young man in the cabin at the headquarters, climb into the rental car, turn on the heat, and know I was two hours away from a hot shower and a bed with blankets. You can't tell I felt guilty because my son wasn't going to get any of that anytime soon. You can't tell how well I slept that night, knowing James was safe, believing there was a plan, understanding what my homework was in terms of finding him a halfway house to go to after he left Nature Quest. You can't tell from looking that I always loved a plan.

You can't tell from looking because all of the pictures in this book are of James. There are no pictures of my visit. And even if there were, you can't tell much from looking.

ALLIANCE HOUSE

APRIL 2013

"He's a bad bet," John, the director of Alliance House, the sober living community in Portland, Maine, explained on the phone. He reiterated what Mike had told us in the woods of Utah about the danger of James relapsing. "He can't go back to Baltimore," John said flatly. "The first twenty-four hours after rehab is the most likely time a person in recovery will relapse. He's been sober for exactly twelve weeks." John went on to remind us that James had never hit "rock bottom." He had never been homeless and was never hungry, penniless, destitute, or in jail. The chances of him relapsing were high. Despite those odds, or maybe because we could pay and were willing to get him to Alliance House from Utah in twenty-four hours, John took him. But he also warned us, "We have a zero-tolerance policy. If he uses one time, and I don't care what his drug of choice is, he's out."

When I want to beat myself up over how James came to be the way he is, when I feel like burning myself on a hot pan, I touch this moment. It's one of those times I had a choice. Go with my husband to Utah, pick James up from St. George, drive him to the airport, fly with him to Portland, Maine, rent a car, drive him to Alliance House, sleep over in a hotel in Portland, buy James some clothes, sheets, towels, meet the people at Alliance House, hang out there for a day or two, fly back to Baltimore. I tell myself I was teaching third grade; I would have had to get a sub for a week. I tell myself Julia and Nathan were home and I needed to be there for them too. I tell myself Daniel was happy to go, he had a more flexible work schedule, he could do this. Those are my excuses for not flying out to Utah to see James after twelve weeks of wilderness therapy.

My reasons, if I want to bathe in that hot oil, are that I wanted him to just keep moving toward the prize. What was the prize? Going back to college, playing soccer again, being a healthy, happy twenty-something-year-old boy. Maybe it was too hard for me to physically see my son so far off the track that he had a beard from twelve weeks in the wilderness, his hair was down to his chin, and all of his clothes at this point were issued to him by Nature Quest. Maybe I needed someone else to do the dirty work, and once James was cleaned up, back on some track, even if it wasn't the one I had in mind, I would be out to visit him. Yes, when I want to pour that guilt over me like maple syrup, I think like this about the time Daniel flew to Utah to do the hard work without me.

I have spent plenty of time with our children without him; he seemed to always be traveling for work when one child or another wound up in the emergency room for stitches, a broken arm, or once, an abscess in the mouth.

But this is a time he did it for me.

ONE HUNDRED MEETINGS IN ONE HUNDRED DAYS

JULY 2012

Pride, when it's an addiction, can be a dangerous emotion. I was seldom without the sound of my father's voice on repeat in the back of my mind, and growing up, I had been willing to give up parts of myself in order to impress him. I knew what made him proud of me: academic excellence, stoicism, sending my children to religious school, having them Bar and Bat Mitzvahed, and achieving professional success, which, in his case, meant master's degrees and well-paying, white-collar jobs. Pride in my own children became a craving for me like food; I needed to satisfy the cravings.

But what of this child? How could I feel pride in this one who bled off the pages of my father's carefully inked story, passed down to me through gulps of amniotic fluid, of how to act, what to say, where to go to college, and what success should look and feel like? No matter that he left college in the middle of his sophomore year, that he was a soccer recruit cut from a college team, that, at this point, he may never graduate college, and that he had cost us thousands of dollars that were never intended for rehab programs. At this moment, I realized that just as there were many ways to make it around that playing board my father so carefully placed me on, pride in this child was going to look like safely making it around the board, passing Go, and collecting two hundred dollars.

I thought I felt something like pride as James held open the door of the First Parish Universalist Church and Daniel and I walked down the steps to the basement, where we joined him in one of his hundred meetings of his first hundred days at Alliance House.

Considering how warm the July day had been in Portland, it was cool in the basement. We found three metal chairs in the semicircle of the seating arrangement. I was surprised at how many people were in this room at 7:30 on a Friday evening; clearly, James was not alone, and neither was I. Next to our meeting room, there was a smaller room with a folding table, coffee, paper cups, and chocolate chip cookies in an open, blue Chips Ahoy bag.

I glanced over at James and smiled at him. He raised his eyebrows up and down and smiled back at me. I almost didn't recognize the feeling in myself, but there it was, bubbling up, raising my chin, making my eyes glisten. He looked healthy, fit, and strong again, a glimmer in his eyes and an easy, playful smile. This kind of pride felt different. I was not sitting at an Ivy League college graduation or cheering for him at a college soccer game. I was not patting him on the back for accepting a triple-figure job offer. No, my pride for this child would not look like that—maybe ever. I told myself to remember that what James had accomplished was a thousand times more difficult than moving in circles around the game board. That path was worn and trodden. The win at the end of that game was one I knew well—the one I had been taught was the endgame. It looked like graduate degrees, home ownership, ski vacations, and private schools. The path James was walking now, unfamiliar and uncertain as it was, forced me to keep rubbing the family stain from my brain and going along for the ride with James. I loved this kid with everything I had. Scrubbing the stain from the grooves of my fingerprints was painful, and who knows if I could ever completely wash it out, but sitting here, hands gripping the seat of my gray, folding metal chair between James and Daniel, I knew I needed to try.

A silence gradually spread over the room. We took turns reading different lines from the promises of AA that we held in our hands on a worn piece of paper.

Daniel read, "We are going to know a new freedom and a new happiness."

James read, "We will not regret the past nor wish to shut the door on it."

I read, "We will know peace." Would I recognize peace if it were spread out before me like still water at sunrise? Would I accept peace if it were gifted to me, wrapped in smooth, brown paper, tied up with soft twine? Would he ever be enough for me?

More silence.

"I'm James," my son said.

I knew his voice despite my eyes being closed. This voice was clear and sure. He was telling me who he was. For God's sake, hear him. Meet him halfway in this room full of strangers. Recognize what he has accomplished and take pride in how he journeyed to this basement in Portland. I was trying out new detergents and scouring the stain with different soaps. It felt different and raw, compromising in a way, but I wanted to set myself free and feel proud of James.

"Hi, James," the entire room responded in unison.

"I'm a recovering addict."

Tears streamed down my face. I opened my eyes and listened to my son tell the group how many weeks he had remained sober, how this week had gone, and what he was grateful for. For the first time, maybe ever in his whole life, I felt like I could love him for who he was, not for how well he lived up to my expectations. He had said, "I'm James." It seems obvious, I know, but this time I believed him. He wasn't James the jokester, James the soccer star, James the Colorado College student. He wasn't Daniel Sherman's son at Friends School, or Judy Sandler's son, the athlete. I heard him. He said he was James Sherman, and he was standing in an AA meeting in the basement of a church in Portland, Maine, and I loved him for it. I hadn't written this script for him, nor could I promise him a happy ending. I understood now I had lost control of my story for him. I dropped the pen and had to resist the urge to pick it up and start writing again.

Even if I started to write a happy ending, it would have been a fairy tale to his real-life story. Because no one, not doctors, friends, teachers, or therapists ever spoke of seeing signs of mental illness in James. Of course, we asked ourselves why James was self-medicating, but the answers that made sense at the time had to do with genetics, stress, peer pressure, and how James chose to entertain himself. We had no reason to suspect an underlying illness, an itch he had to scratch until it bled, anxiety and fear so powerful they rolled like a tsunami inside him.

If James's substance use disorder in his adolescent years was a symptom of mental illness that would be diagnosed in his mid-twenties, I missed it like butter on a shelf in the refrigerator. It could be that I was only looking for a specific brand of butter. I was focused on exactly what that package looked like—substance use disorder. I recognized its signs and understood the possible roots of the disease. True to my nature, I identified the problem, did everything in my power to "fix it," and after James had proven himself "cured," I thought we were all ready to "keep a-goin'." While I acknowledged substance use disorder in James for the stubborn disease it is, I did not unearth mental illness as the root. Was I looking hard enough? Even now, in retrospect, mental illness seems like something that was invisible in James until it wasn't. That part of him was like writing with invisible ink, imperceptible until you drip the drops of magic on the writing. I would have sworn it wasn't there. Doctors and psychologists tell me the early use of drugs can trigger bipolar disorder later in a person's life. But they also tell me underlying bipolar disease can cause substance abuse. I'll never know.

Mental illness would eventually crash over James, but that night at the AA meeting, it just looked like butter, and I felt like we had it all wrapped up.

TSUNAMI

DECEMBER 2016

One minute, all is well, and the next, you better be prepared to duck, pivot, or keep going. Life with James taught me to do all three at once but not necessarily in that order. In December 2016, I was driving to work at school when my cell phone rang. I flipped it over on the front seat to see who it was. I knew I shouldn't talk and drive, but the caller ID read "James," so I answered the call.

"Good morning, bud. What's up?" It wasn't a good sign that he was calling me at 7:30 on a weekday morning. My fear of phone calls had somewhat subsided since James's teenage years. Once I experienced a call from the police or from a concerned teacher, there was little rest for my brain; I was on high alert for years. It wasn't a question of when James would return safely home in the evenings; it was a question of if I was going to hear from a hospital, or if the police were going to appear at our door. When James entered Nature Quest Wilderness Therapy in Utah, and then Alliance House in Maine, I was able to breathe, to settle into more of a routine. It was like walking on a pond I knew was frozen; I didn't have to worry if my next step would plunge me into freezing water. I had faith in John, the director of Alliance House, and his staff. But most importantly, I had faith in James that he wanted to stay sober. At twenty-four years old, he was living and working as a recreational therapist at Oceanside Psychiatric Hospital, having graduated from the University of Southern Maine with a degree in recreational therapy. He lived in a house in Portland, Maine, with three friends from Alliance House.

The ring of a telephone will always trigger panic in me, particularly when I see it's James calling. But during the few years James spent at wilderness therapy and Alliance House, I experienced some relief. For the first time in a long time, when friends asked about my children, I could honestly report they were all doing well. I don't believe I was naive to feel we might have been finding our way out of the maze with James. He seemed to be figuring it out for himself, getting his map stamped as he cleared his own path. It's not that I didn't see it coming. There was nothing to see.

Or, I was so relieved to be back on the "normal" setting, I just pressed the button, turned around, and trusted the machine would do what it was supposed to do.

This phone call interrupted the cycle.

"Mom, I need to talk to you." He sounded panicked and scared. "I know what you and Dad did for me in high school."

I thought for a second this was one of the twelve steps of AA, making amends with your parents. But then there was more.

"I am remembering that I killed someone," he said. His voice was slow, like he was explaining a dream to me. "Like in eleventh or twelfth grade, and you and Dad hired a lawyer, and you made it all go away. I think I caused a car accident and I killed someone in the accident."

I listened to him as I turned into the school driveway, past the blacktop playground and the grassy field where James played football with his friends in elementary school. This voice sounded like James, but nothing he was telling me made sense. I felt like I was checking out at the grocery store and the cashier had just told me my total was $250,000. What? My body froze in the driver's seat. My mouth was open, but I didn't know what to say.

"So I just wanted you to know I did that. And whatever I should do now to make up for that, I am ready to do it. It's like now I know what I was meant to do. I feel a strong connection to everyone, and I just want to help them."

I pulled into the lower school parking lot but did not attempt to get out of the car. Around me, children stumbled out of cars with their backpacks tossed over their shoulders while their parents shouted after them, "Have a good day! Love you!" I closed my eyes in the car, thought about my next move, and tried hard not to panic.

I kept my voice calm. "James, is someone with you right now? Because I have to tell you that you are not making sense. You never killed anyone in a car crash. You may have hidden a lot from us in high school, but that is something Dad and I would have found out. It didn't happen. I assure you, James. That did not happen."

The whole time I was saying this, I was wondering if it *had* actually happened. Was it possible James *was* in a drunk driving accident, that someone died, and we never knew about it? *No,* I reassured myself, *you are making sense*. James was not.

"I gotta go, Mom. But we can talk more later. I just wanted to let you know I remember all that happened to me." He sounded calm, like he was strangely under control, when in fact, he had just ignited a pile of dry leaves.

"Don't hang up, James." I needed to know where he was and what he was going to do next. I wasn't sure I would be able to get out of the car if I didn't hear some kind of reassurance that he was only temporarily off-kilter and would go to work and we could settle this later in the evening.

But he did hang up.

The silence that followed marked the beginning of a disconnect that I still struggle to bridge with James. He probably doesn't divide his life into a before and after, and if he does, it's likely before sobriety and after. But to me, there exists a James before this phone call, and a different James after this phone call. One therapist advised me to grieve the James I knew before the phone call, like a death. I prefer to keep striking the match because I know the James I remember is still there. I will meet him where he is, over and over again, until the wind stops blowing and the flame burns by itself.

Where did he go?

At lunchtime, I checked my phone again, and there was a message from his girlfriend, Jessica, saying, "James is safe. We are in St. Mark's Psychiatric Emergency Room. Call me when you can."

I was relieved to hear the message, but something about the word "safe" was having the opposite effect of reassurance. I watched the gray dot on my voicemail slide to its end. Twelve seconds. That's all it took to tell me my son was in a psychiatric hospital in Maine while I sat in a booth in a school cafeteria surrounded by the loud banter and laughter of small children happily gnawing on barbecue chicken wings, their fingers brown and oily.

The normal setting on the washing machine? It just clicked off, and an error code took its place, flashing silent red lights. I went into a well-rehearsed mode of anesthetized and robotic.

I would need to tell my small students to wash their hands before they ran off to recess.

CARRY ON

I am my father's daughter, and I learned his lessons all too well; carry on, keep a-goin'. And so, I did. I was good at compartmentalizing. I wanted to keep my job. I had two other children, classes to teach, and at 3:30 that afternoon, a carpool line to direct. There was dinner to cook later and a dog to walk and feed. But I wonder now what would have happened had I allowed myself to feel the pain of those words: "James is safe."

What if I had cried instead of going numb, as was my habit?

What if I had said aloud in that school cafeteria booth, "Oh my god, I have to go," darted out of the cafeteria, sprinted to my classroom, grabbed my pocketbook and keys, and left my colleagues midbite, holding their forks in the air?

I would have been able to say, "I was there for you."

I would have been able to say, "I did all I could do for you."

I know none of that would have cured my son, but it may have helped me in the way that showing up and confronting the hard stuff always feels better in the long run. Somewhere in that moment, I knew what I was doing. I made a choice, maybe a subconscious choice, an aimless choice—definitely one I regret.

I felt guilty about opening car doors at carpool that afternoon, smiling and waving goodbye to other people's children instead of sitting at St. Mark's Hospital in Lewiston, Maine, with my own son.

I still do.

PHONE CALL TO ST. MARK'S HOSPITAL

LEWISTON, MAINE, DECEMBER 2016

Whenever I tried to call James on the hall phone at St. Mark's, he never answered.

Someone else was always on the other end. I wonder if he was as uncomfortable talking to me from St. Mark's psychiatric ward as I was talking to him from the comfort of my home.

"James Sherman? Yeah, I know him. Hold on, let me see if I can find him." The seconds felt like minutes until footsteps approached.

"Hello?" It was James, just a subdued rendering of himself.

I paced the length of our house from the family room through the living room, across the dining room to a sunroom. Then I turned around and walked the same path back in the other direction. "Hey, bud, it's me. How's it going?" Kind of a desperate question, I was aware, but I had to start somewhere.

"Hey, Mom. It's going. You know, I'm okay. I think I'm gonna be here for a week or two. They won't let me out yet."

I felt every mile of the distance between us, and from my end, I was grateful. I smelled from our kitchen greasy fried eggs sizzling in a pan. I heard Nathan pouring steaming hot coffee into a mug. It made me think about how James was not in the middle of his familiar routine right now, about how he was completely out of his comfort zone. Maybe he was inhaling the scent of wax from polished linoleum floors, or the sweet odor of small, overcooked sausages offered to him for breakfast on a pale-peach plastic tray. What kind of mother is secretly grateful to be hundreds of miles away from her son who is passing his days behind the locked doors of a psychiatric floor? What kind of mother is satisfied with this check-in from afar, this show of concern that neither James nor I could touch or feel? This kind of mother. This kind of mother had been taught—in fact, persuaded—that boundaries like the one I was drawing between James and me were better for both of us. This kind of mother grew up with the understanding that fears created conflict, and conflict made for feelings, and it was safer and less painful not to feel. It was easy to convince myself, and my husband, that James was in good hands, that we could only see him for a few hours a day anyway, that being there wasn't going to change anything. And that might have been true for James, but years later, it wasn't true for me.

"That's okay, bud. Stay until you feel stable. Let them get some medication worked out. Let the doctors figure out what happened." Easy for me to say as I sat down at the family room table and scanned the headlines of the *New York Times*. It was unclear to me if James even understood or remembered why Jessica had taken him to St. Mark's.

"Yeah, I'm on some meds now. Not exactly sure what I'm taking, though."

"That's okay. We can figure it out. Have you spent time with a doctor?" I wanted details, names, and a diagnosis. My mind was relentlessly spreading the stain: name the disease, get the treatment, return to work and your friends, your home in Portland, and your girlfriend. Since he was over twenty-one, no doctor would talk to us until James signed a release form. Our only source of information was James, and he wasn't proving to be informative. I needed specifics in order to pretend I had some kind of control about getting James out of St. Mark's and back to his life as a recreational therapist. But pretending would be what I was doing, because what kind of mother believes she can help her son recover from a delusional episode from hundreds of miles away?

"I guess so. I think I did. Yeah, I spoke to a doctor yesterday. I think some friends are coming to visit tomorrow. That'll be good."

"That's great! I'm glad they are coming to see you." I clung to any fragment of normalcy from the outside world that would walk through the doors of the psychiatric unit at St. Mark's. Maybe his friends would be a reliable source of information. At least they were showing up, unlike his mother. They offered me yet another reason to stay home. He had visitors, friends, and doctors.

"You need anything, James?" I asked from the safety of my family room. "Not sure if I am allowed to send you anything, but I can talk to your friends and have them bring you something."

"Nah, I'm good. Nothing to bring. I love you, Mom. I gotta go."

"Love you too, bud. We'll call you tomorrow." I was left midpace in the family room, holding the cell phone, staring out the window at the empty bird feeders and frozen ferns on the hill that separated our house from the road.

Looking back, my decision to stay in Baltimore while James was checked into St. Mark's was probably the best example of what my father had taught me so well. It was a real-life lesson playing out the way he would have handled it. And I even had the words to persuade Daniel to stay home. "He's twenty-five years old," I reasoned with my husband. "He's going to have to learn to recognize his symptoms, take his medication, and ask for help." Staying home and pretending to control the situation from our cell phones was much easier. There would be no buzzing outside heavy metal doors to see my son, no sleepless nights in hotel beds, no restaurant food three meals a day, no searching of James's deep eyes to find the truth of how he was doing. I was convinced he would do as the doctors prescribed, be released from the hospital, and get back to himself, the way he was before the phone call when he informed me he had killed someone.

Three days into his ten-day stay at St. Mark's, James signed a release allowing Daniel and me to speak with his doctors. Over the next week, during half-hour scheduled phone calls, we learned that while working at Oceanside Psychiatric Hospital, James had been unable to maintain an appropriate therapeutic distance from his patients and was taking on the life events of his patients. James believed he had committed the same crimes as one of his patients, which included killing someone in a car accident and leaving the scene. James related to the doctor that Daniel and I had helped him cover up his crime by hiring a lawyer. The next words out of the psychiatrist's mouth were, "Our team has diagnosed James with bipolar type II disorder."

Hearing the words might have been shocking or life-changing had we not swum this far with James. As it was, the diagnosis felt like the doctor had just torn a bigger hole in our bag and we could shake the dirt out. What happened to James had a name, a treatment, and a prognosis. Talking to the doctor at St. Mark's was not nearly as frightening to me as hearing James tell me that he thought he had killed someone in a car accident. Whereas I felt the need to file that incident away and move on with my day, I could hear the words this doctor was saying and let them drop on me like a slow drizzle, soaking me with the idea that James had a mental illness. If James's phone call was the electrical storm that sent me running, this was the clearing. I was beginning to understand it was going to be impossible to love James as he was if I didn't dilute this family stain. I couldn't help him come back to himself if I didn't accept that mental illness was going to be my stepchild.

In a way, everything, but also nothing, changed when James was released from St. Mark's. Part of me wanted to believe James would swallow his new pills, go back to work at Oceanside, and everything would return to normal. And yet, now that he had been diagnosed with bipolar type II disorder, I felt like the doctor had placed a band-aid on my son. We were told the longer he stayed on the lithium, the better his chances were of not having a repeat episode. In this murky land of mental illness, even if he took the lithium, I wondered if his delusions would return.

FROM JAMES'S APPLICATION TO COMPASS ROSE

Deep Healing Without Meds

JULY 2020

I began working at Oceanside Psychiatric Center approximately four years after graduating from USM. I was in a relationship with an LPN I worked with and continued my external seeking for validation of being ok with myself by cheating on my girlfriend, I then began working for St Mark's after resigning from Oceanside for "personal reasons." During the time I was on administrative leave, I attended a Native American Church ceremony with a friend who was a previous patient and who described himself as having housing challenges and was living on the streets by choice, defining homelessness as "waiting in endless lines." During my third year working at Oceanside Psychiatric Center as a recreational therapist, I was hospitalized in Lewiston, Maine for thinking I killed someone in a drunk driving accident and thinking I was a sacred clown and not eating or sleeping as well. This elevated state of consciousness was brought about by being prescribed Effexor by my primary care physician and doing pranayama practices daily.

NO MORE MEDS

JULY 2019

It wasn't difficult for me to conclude that James had stopped taking the lithium. On the medication, he seemed content to sit for long periods of time, something not characteristic of the loud, animated, and impulsive James I knew growing up in our house. But with the lithium came stability. His thoughts were ordered and predictable in a way that I found reassuring. James was different now at this "after the call" period, but so was I. Scared straight, shaken out to what really mattered to me most, all I wished for James now was for him to be happy and to be able to live independently. I was proud of the progress he had made in the past year; he was seven years sober, working as a recreational therapist in a psychiatric hospital, and active in AA. From time to time, I would hear that one of his friends was in medical school, another living in New York, working in finance. As long as James was sober, stable, and supporting himself with a job he enjoyed, I stood tall and content. But like a lot of decisions James made, it didn't matter how I felt. Because apparently, James had other thoughts about taking the medication.

When he arrived for a visit at our lake house in July, I met him in the driveway and watched him climb out of his car. He gave me a hug and held on to me for what felt like a few seconds too long. "Love you, Mom," he said, unprompted. This was my first clue. On medication, he would have skipped the hug and walked slowly to the front door with me.

He reached into the back seat of his Toyota 4Runner and pulled out a drum. "You like it? I made it myself. It's bent cedar and elk hide. I'm working on the drumsticks. I'm gonna try to finish them up here this weekend." His eyes had a shiny glint I hadn't seen in a while. In general, the lithium dulled James's expressions and slowed his motions. When he was on lithium, his step was deliberate and his movements were slightly less coordinated, considering his athleticism.

Carrying his drum and drumsticks, he followed me into the house. He had no backpack, no sign of a change of clothing, toothbrush, or bathing suit. He sat down on the sofa in the family room, the sun still a cool orange blur visible behind the trees and houses across the lake, the water a flat mirror. This was Mother Nature demonstrating her indifference to me, showing me what an insignificant speck I was in her plan for the day. James placed the drum between his knees, took a deep breath, and tapped the stretched elk hide lightly, alternating beats between his hands. He closed his eyes and found his rhythm.

"James," I said, after a minute of steady beating. "Stop. I can't deal with the drumming at this hour of the morning. Want some coffee? Dad just made some." Daniel sat at the table, looking straight at me with wide eyes.

James stopped his hands on the drums. "No thanks, I'm off caffeine. Have any decaf tea?"

I had plenty of herbal tea in the pantry, but I felt like, at that moment, we needed to address a large elephant in the room. My chest was tight as I tried to pull in air, my eyes narrowed, and a wave of frustration crept across my face and settled in my hands. I had to do something with my hands. If James was off his medication, an episode of delusional thoughts, unpredictable behavior, and panicked phone calls to us from his friends could not be far behind. I had worked hard to override my father's voice in my head. But it seemed to me that James needed to hold up his end of the couch, and it felt like he had just dropped it.

"Sure," I said. "I have decaf tea in the pantry. Come over here and pick out what kind you want."

James placed his drum on the floor and, with a little too much spring in his step, walked over to the closet in the kitchen. He paused before sliding the door open and glanced up at me standing at the sink. "Thanks, Mom."

He grinned like he had found a hundred-dollar bill on the shelf in the closet instead of a box of herbal tea.

I couldn't stop myself. "James, I'm glad you came up this weekend. I know this sounds strange, but you seem a little different. Like a little too happy? You know, the drums, the affection, the smiles? I mean, it's all good but just different than the last time I saw you. Anything changed with you?"

Daniel sat at the table, his eyes on his laptop, but I knew his ears were on this conversation. Then he looked up from the screen and watched James pull a green box of organic peppermint tea from the pantry. Daniel's eyes followed James as he took out a tea bag, walked over to the teapot on the stove, popped open the silver top, and filled it with cold water from the sink. He placed the teapot on the stove, turned the burner on low, and smiled at me again like I wasn't speaking the same language as him, like he wished he could understand what I was saying but he just couldn't.

"What's up, James? You want to tell us something?" Daniel obviously saw the same elephant I had spotted.

"Yeah, I guess I should tell you that I decided to stop taking lithium. It's a very dangerous drug, did you know that? I mean, it's bad for your kidneys, it makes me have tremors. It's really not good for you to be on lithium long term, did you know that?"

I had been waiting for James to say exactly what he'd just said, and yet, I didn't have a response. Not only had he dropped his end of the sofa, but he also had no plans to try to pick it up again. I didn't care anymore where he placed the sofa. I just needed him to support his end. My stomach dropped, and a hollow feeling took its place.

James filled the silence with more words. "Do you know the side effects of lithium? I went off the drug because I hated the way I was on it. That's not the way I want to live my life. Besides, are you aware that Western medicine is in bed with pharmaceutical companies? That the more lithium prescriptions my doctor writes, the more money the drug companies make?"

"Well, hold on, James," Daniel said, calmly pushing his laptop out of the way so he could have a clear view of James standing at the kitchen counter, sipping his tea. "First, you have a psychiatrist who you trust. At least, we assumed you did, as you have been seeing him for a year now. Don't you think Dr. Gordon has your best interest in mind when he prescribes the medication?

It's not quite that simple, James. Yes, drug companies make money when people buy the drugs. But that doesn't mean you don't need the medication. It's been working pretty well for you for a year now."

I shook my head and sat down at the table next to Daniel and agreed with him that this was a trade-off we were willing to make with the pharmaceutical companies.

James placed his mug on the counter and took steps toward the table but stopped and did not sit in a chair. His voice was loud, his hands animated. "It hasn't been working, and how would you know since you aren't on it? I don't like the way it makes me feel. I've been off of it for a few weeks now, and I feel great—much better in fact. I'm not taking any medications. This is how I am. I hope you like it."

This was a battle we were not going to win in the next hour, or even over the next few days or years. I looked out the windows stretching across the back of the house. The sun had pooled light on the lake. An occasional fish broke the surface of the water. Daybreak. But now what? Would we debate the pros and cons of treating mental illness with psychopharmaceuticals all weekend?

I tried. I really tried to listen to James's points about how medicine for mental illness is overprescribed, and how the Native Americans and other cultures treat people who see things "differently" as seekers and soothsayers. Why, he asked, couldn't we just see him as "neurodiverse" and accept him just the way he was? I considered his points about the side effects of drugs and how the scientists really didn't know the long-term effects of many medicines used to treat mental illness. All weekend, we listened, nodded, and considered his arguments. But behind closed doors,

Daniel and I felt afraid. We knew we were about to be backed into a corner.

James was an adult. He could do whatever he wanted to do, and we had no power to control whether or not he took his medication. But the truth was, whenever he was off the medication, we took the calls from his friends, from his girlfriend, from the police. In the privacy of our bedroom, Daniel and I said things to one another like, "Go ahead, James, go off the meds. Just don't list us as your emergency contact anymore." We told each other, "He can do what he wants. He's all grown-up. But when he winds up in jail, I'm not coming to bail him out."

And while I knew that was the responsible thing to say, and was, in fact, how the therapists and psychiatrists had suggested we talk to James, actually saying these words made me feel empty and hypocritical. I didn't think I was strong enough to climb into my bed and fall asleep if my son was lying in a jail cell and money was the only thing between us.

MEKONG ASIAN BISTRO

OCTOBER 2019

I knew I shouldn't drive through Portland at dinner time and not offer to take James to dinner. What kind of mother would do that? And as it turned out, Daniel and I would be driving right through Portland around 6:30 in the evening on our way from Baltimore back to Maine, where we planned to make sure we could survive a Maine winter before we sold our house in Baltimore.

When James made the decision, a few months prior, to stop taking lithium, the settled feeling I held in my body when he was in wilderness, then at Alliance House, and more recently, when he was taking his medication and holding down a job for the last few years, cracked open like a sinkhole.

"It's not your decision, and it's out of your control," my therapist told me. "Separate and allow James to experience the natural consequences of his choices."

The natural consequences of his choices? That looked like homelessness, jail, or life in and out of psychiatric hospitals to me.

Separate? Hard to hang up the phone when his best friend called me and told me that James was not making sense. Where was the line between my need to control how James treated his disease and my ability to let it go? My need to control James's treatment plan was undoubtedly wrapped up in my father's gift he had subtly passed on to me, although I had tried repeatedly to say no thank you. But a voice inside me (was it mine or my father's?) said this time was different. I rationalized that James didn't know what was best for him at this moment. He was in a manic episode, refused to acknowledge the diagnosis, and therefore saw no reason to be treated. Why would I let go of my end of the rope when I knew he was only pretending to hold on to his end?

Taking James to dinner was the right thing to do. I just wasn't sure I had the energy to replay the same conversation with him about the importance of maintaining a routine, looking for a job while he waited out his leave of absence from Oceanside, and our view that medication *and* meditation were important for his mental health. If I had been able to hold a boundary, close the door on my father's voice telling me to stay in control, and listen to the advice of my therapist, Daniel and I would have blown through Portland. But as it was, I felt the need to at least try—try to convince James to take the meds, help him plan, or, as my father would have done, make the plan for him.

"Mom?" His voice was soft and groggy.

"Hey James, yeah, it's Mom. How's it going?"

"I don't know. I mean I'm really tired. I haven't been sleeping. So I was taking a nap. I took a Zyprexa to try to get some sleep."

Outside the window, the smooth white highway stretched out mile after mile. Daniel glanced over at me, frowned, then stared ahead at the road again.

"I'm sorry you haven't been sleeping, James," I said. "You do sound tired. Where did you get the Zyprexa? I'm pretty sure Zyprexa isn't a drug for sleep. It's an antidepressant or antipsychotic. It's not a one-and-done drug for sleep."

"Yeah? Well, I took it. I think I got it from my doctor. Or maybe from Paul. Yeah, I think Paul gave it to me because I can't sleep."

I wished I hadn't heard that. I had to hold myself back from getting into an argument with James about his use of Zyprexa, and about Paul Jackson-Meade's judgment for prescribing it to James for sleep. Paul Jackson-Meade was a graduate of Stanford Medical School, a licensed MD, who, along with his partner, Elizabeth, was interested in what Indigenous cultures had to offer the modern world when it came to psychosis. Together, from their home in Orono, Maine, they ran a counseling practice based on how psychotherapy can be modified to include insights into traditional healing. James and his current girlfriend, Isabella, had visited them frequently for Native American Church ceremonies, sweat lodges, and Native Institute workshops. I felt helpless in the face of what I believed was James's misuse of medication.

"How about you wake up, take a shower, and meet Dad and me at Saigon for dinner? I think we should be there around 6:00."

Silence.

I heard breathing.

"Okay, okay. I can do that. I'll see you there."

"Good, see you in a little while. Saigon, right?"

But he was gone. Hopefully not back to sleep.

We drove past the restaurant, but it was dark inside, and the neon sign in the window read, "Closed." We had forgotten it was Sunday evening. I saw James's car in the parking lot, and I could barely make out his figure in the driver's seat. He was staring at his phone. I tapped on his window and he startled, then unrolled his window and looked at me.

"It's closed," he announced, pointing his head toward the building. "I forgot; they're closed on Sundays."

"I see that."

A dog barked in the distance, and the streetlamps cast murky light onto the pavement.

"You know another place nearby?" I wasn't leaving him in the dark, obsessed with his phone, in the parking lot. I felt deeply worried and not about to separate or depart. He may not have wanted our help that night, but he looked like he needed it. I was in "go" mode, "here's what we're going to do, James" mode, and I was hungry.

"How about that Thai place across the street? It's pretty good, and we can park here," James suggested. He turned off his engine and stepped out of the car, but he never let go of his phone, even as we walked across the parking lot and crossed the street to Mekong Asian Bistro.

The restaurant was empty, which is never a good sign, even on a Sunday night.

A young woman arrived at our table and wiped down the speckled Formica square with a wet cloth that I could only hope had not been used to wipe multiple tables before ours. I will never know. She handed us three sticky, plastic menus.

I can't remember what I ordered; I just remember what it looked like. In a steaming pale yellow broth, overcooked beige noodles sank to the bottom of the white bowl. Cubes of orange carrots bobbed in the broth, and bits of overcooked broccoli floated away from their stems. I glanced up at Daniel; his eyes were getting that watery glisten to them right before he cries. A wave of nausea crept up my throat. I shook my head ever so slightly at Daniel.

Don't cry, I was trying to tell him, *and please don't walk out of this restaurant*.

What James told us that evening became one with my memory of that soup. His words, the salty yellow broth, the frozen, thawing vegetables, the soggy noodles—it's all one floating image for me.

"I haven't really been sleeping. I really need to sleep." He put his head in his hands, his elbows on the table.

"So you said," Daniel replied quietly, trying to get James to look at him.

James stared into his plate of chicken pad thai but made no attempt to eat. He held his phone tightly in one hand, and with the other hand, his fork pushed the gluey noodles around the plate. "I went to this Native American Church ceremony at Paul and Elizabeth's. It was like a healing thing. And I took peyote; it was part of the ceremony, you know? But I haven't slept since I got back. So Paul prescribed Zyprexa for sleep. But I haven't slept for more than a few hours in like a week."

James looked up and stared at Daniel and me, his eyes watery and dull.

So many questions ran through my mind. I wanted to ask him if he still considered himself sober, having taken peyote as part of a ceremony. And when was the last time he had attended an AA meeting? Was he eating regularly? Had he spoken to anyone lately, like within the last twenty-four hours? When did he last change his clothes?

But I knew better than to fire these kinds of questions at him now.

"How can we help you, James?" This was one of the nonthreatening, purposeful questions I had been advised to ask James in situations like this, when I felt like I wanted to break down and sob.

James looked at us through glassy eyes. "Can I come back to the lake house with you? I just need some sleep. I need some love, some warmth, you know?"

These words from my son seemed innocent enough, the kind that would make any mother's heart bleed. But with these words, I felt like James backed me into a corner, and I was stuck. I had no choice but to fight or give in. Continue the family rule and believe against all odds that I could take over and make him well by providing him with love, warmth, and sleep, or I could wipe the stain clean and tell him no. *No, James, I don't know. But I do know that love and warmth don't usually alleviate a bipolar episode.* It had been a little over four months since James had stopped taking lithium, and in that time, he'd lost his job, taken a leave of absence from another job, and become delusional. What I wanted to ask James was how he thought this was all going for him. I wanted to tell him that I felt love and warmth for him when he took medication. I wanted to whisper quietly but directly to him and tell him I didn't believe in shamans or Native American Church ceremonies to heal his brain. And I wanted to make it clear to him that I believed his brain needed healing.

Instead, maybe because I could not trust James to heal himself, and I would not let him go to suffer the consequences that would have taken him over that night, I said to James, "You can come back to Lincolnville with us. After dinner, we'll follow you to your house so you can get some clothes, whatever else you need."

James nodded slowly and looked at me. He said, "That's okay. I don't really need anything from my house. Let's just go."

SEEKING ADVICE

NOVEMBER 2021

The word "cult" felt increasingly appropriate to me to describe the group of people who had James's attention. The cult included Isabella, his new girlfriend, Paul and Elizabeth, and social media sites like Resistance Recovery, Mad in America, and Madness Radio. I felt he was drowning in sweat lodges and worshipping therapists like Henry Reed whose life mission it was to "free" people from psychiatric drugs. James could be different, he could call himself neurodiverse, but I believed in science and a line, albeit a fuzzy one, between sane and psychotic. I wasn't willing yet to "lose" the battle; losing would look like James floating from sweat lodges to meditation retreats, and witnessing him taking drops of homeopathic medicines while plugged into Resistance Recovery. If I had seen improvement in his mental health, motivation to support himself, thoughts that were ordered and made sense, and some semblance of executive functioning skills, I may have been more willing to join his cult. But his cult leaders were nowhere in sight when he was asked to take a leave of absence from his job or when he spoke of people tapping his phone, and of photographs that called out to him from the walls. One could argue his cult members were allowing him to suffer the natural consequences of his behavior and that when he hit rock bottom, he would have some epiphany about how to heal himself. But what if he didn't have an epiphany? What if he had damaged his brain function by abusing drugs in his adolescence? What if, as I had been reading about, delusions caused more delusions, and that the longer he remained untreated, the longer he would remain in a bipolar episode? Call me a control freak, call me a mother—this was too painful to watch. Not to mention that James was, at this very moment, by his request and our permission, sheltering in our house. I needed help, advice from the experts, a map with no alternate routes to follow. I wanted to be on a strict diet. If you told me the results would be successful, that my son would regain some semblance of his former self, I swear I would not cheat. Just tell me what to eat.

Daniel and I made an appointment with Dr. Glenn Treisman, a leading specialist in bipolar disorder at Johns Hopkins Hospital. Because we were living through a worldwide pandemic, the appointment took place over Zoom, and we were granted half an hour with him. When Dr. Treisman appeared on Daniel's laptop on our kitchen table in Maine, he looked to be about my age, maybe a little younger, in his late fifties, with salt-and-pepper hair. Dressed casually in a button-down shirt and comfortable brown sweater, he had a sincere smile that he wasn't afraid to use, and even though we were staring at each other on computer screens, hundreds of miles away, I felt certain he was listening. Daniel talked first and gave Dr. Treisman a brief history of James's substance abuse and his bipolar diagnosis. He mentioned that James was now eight years sober, and Dr. Treisman's brown eyes softened. He got a little misty-eyed and said, "Ahh, I love to hear that. My son is living with addiction issues. Sorry, go on." Daniel continued and told him that what we most needed to hear was advice on how to get James back on the medication that seemed to be working for him but that he had stopped taking and that he refused, for various philosophical reasons, to begin taking again.

Dr. Treisman nodded and allowed for a moment of silence.

"Let me ask you something," he said. "If your son were a heroin addict, would you be feeding the den?" His eyes looked back at us with raised eyebrows and his mouth closed, waiting for our answer.

I was uncomfortable with the pause and filled it with words that I could only hope were true. "I'm sure not."

"Well, it's the same thing. Your son has a disease. There's a biological basis for the disease. By giving him money and supporting him and his current habits, you are feeding his beliefs. He doesn't need to change his behavior. He can stay with this girl, wallow in his illness, and accuse everyone else of being crazy."

"I guess that's true," I said, unconvinced that I was making James sicker by supporting him financially. I don't know how to sever this particular tie in my relationship with my son, and if I need to let him bleed out, I am going to need some anesthesia and a blindfold. I still believe I have the power to save him if only I can force the pills down his throat. I still believe it's in his best interest for me to save him by controlling how he treats his illness. And that may be true, but what I didn't realize at this point is that, like his substance use disorder, only James can help James. Before this call with Dr. Treisman, I would not have been convinced that no amount of money, arguing, threatening, tough love, or love would enable me to control James. Nothing would work. But I didn't know that yet.

"The hardest part of understanding someone who is bipolar is understanding that they do not see themselves as sick. Nothing is wrong with them. Everyone else has suddenly turned against them. It's called anosognosia. It's caused by physical changes to the brain, and it's the reason for James's lack of insight into his own illness." Dr. Treisman spoke with an authority that I needed to hear. His words quieted the deafening noise in my brain. I needed to hear the words "biological basis" in describing James's behavior. I took comfort in the label "anosognosia." It was like he had picked up my little car from the floor and placed it back on the Hot Wheels track.

"He needs to be on the drugs that have been proven to work for bipolar disorder. That's it. It's highly unlikely he will get better without the medication."

We spoke to Dr. Treisman for much longer than our half-hour appointment. We discussed how to commit someone to Hopkins; he gave us the names of five other doctors he would recommend. He assured us that if we wanted to get James to Baltimore, he would monitor his case. He told us to call him anytime, and he gave us his cell phone number. I didn't want to hang up, as if disconnecting from him would drain the certainty out of my renewed sense of self. I knew what I had to do, and if it didn't work, I would need to find the strength to remove the blindfold, let myself run out of anesthesia, and let James clean up the blood.

I wanted James to talk to Dr. Treisman so badly that I could feel it in my gut. Chalk it up to one more thing I didn't have control over. In fact, when I had the opportunity to tell James over a

Zoom call with him and his therapist, Henry Reed about this great Hopkins doctor who was willing to talk to him, James held up his thumb, raised his eyebrows in a sarcastic look of glee, and said, "Cool, Mom."

THINKING OUT OF THE BOX

JUNE 2020

The person I was in Maine crept up on me, and I liked her. I could walk around the town of Camden, stop at Lincolnville General Store for a slice of pizza, pick up toilet paper and dish soap at Hannafords, and not one person knew who I was. I felt no pressure up there to be who I was in Baltimore. I didn't want to teach anymore, and I loved sitting down to write every morning. I had completed an MFA in creative nonfiction, and if I had dreams of publishing my work, they were my dreams, not my father's. Maine felt bigger to me than Baltimore; I felt like I had been let out of a box. I had never bothered to open the flaps of the box to consider living somewhere else. I was born in Baltimore and raised there. I married a Baltimore boy in Baltimore, and we raised our family ten miles from my childhood home. My parents grew up in neighborhoods just outside of Baltimore, married in my mother's childhood home, and raised my brother, sister, and me in Mt. Washington, in Baltimore City. My roots in Baltimore were deep and firmly embedded. I never doubted that I would live out my life and die in Baltimore. But when James checked into Alliance House in Portland, Maine, and Daniel decided to partially retire from his career in finance and began to make the drive from Baltimore to Rockport, Maine, to attend photography workshops at Maine Media Workshops, I spent increasing amounts of time at our house on the lake in Lincolnville. I discovered I had not forgotten what my mother and grandmother taught me about fishing, and my mind and body, usually speeding along, remained still for long periods of time while I sat on the dock or in a small boat waiting for a bite. Maybe because I didn't know or care who I was up here, I was more flexible about trying new things. Ice fishing? Cross-country skiing? A drive up the coast to explore another town, visit the Bowdoin Museum, or try for my captain's license? Never in any of my thoughts and plans for my future did I imagine myself leaving the field of education, moving to Maine, and rethinking who and how I wanted to be. I gave myself permission to drop the control, expectations, and stain of my father's plan for us all at the Maryland state border. My children were adulting now, the youngest about to graduate from college. For the first time in close to twenty-five years, I allowed myself to think about me. What did I want to be when I grew up, or old? Where did I want to go, now that I didn't have to be at Friends School, teaching at 7:30 every morning? What would be my routine, and how would I spend my days? I wasn't sure, but I liked the sound of the questions, and I was planning to protect my new freedom.

SYNCHRONICITY

JUNE 2020

I didn't realize how much I loved living in Maine, and how protective I was of my space and my new routine, until James visited us one weekend in late June of 2020. He stepped over some invisible boundary I buried around everything I loved up there, and I forgot to tell him about it.

It was a Saturday morning, after some coffee. I asked James if he wanted to walk the dog with me on the trail that looped around the pond. He said he would like that, and I grabbed a leash for the dog and slipped on some tennis shoes.

"You want to borrow a pair of Dad's shoes?" I asked because he was barefoot.

"No thanks. I'll be barefoot. It's called grounding, Mom."

"What does that mean, James?" It was true that the trail was covered in soft pine needles and it was a warm morning, but there were errant sticker bushes, and occasionally, animals pooped along the trail.

"Grounding means you get closer to the earth, Mom. I am connecting myself to all the electrical activity going on right now. We're not alone, you know? Everything's connected."

"I am aware, James, that we are not alone. And I know that things are connected. But you might cut your foot on a piece of rock or glass, and then you will be connected to Pen Bay Medical Center." I knew exactly what I was doing. I was purposely throwing concrete, practical advice in front of him because I knew he was thinking on another wavelength. Grounding, drumming, meditation, and rhythmic breathing were all possible treatments for James's symptoms of bipolar disorder, but in addition to Western medication. Since our appointment with Dr. Treisman, and my recent promise to myself to make boundaries to protect what I enjoyed in Maine, the line between accepting James's behavior as eccentric, and judging his lifestyle decisions to be irresponsible, was becoming clearer to me. My anger was coming out in the form of sarcasm, which was not new for me, although I rarely used it on my children, and it wasn't a particularly effective way of communicating with James. But reasoning with him—about the need to wear shoes on a walk in the woods, to the more pressing necessity that he take medication—failed to change his behavior in any way. As his mother, I wanted to give him the benefit of my doubt. I did my homework on his preferred treatment plan, and I was willing to shift, to slow down, to meet him where he was currently treading water. But I was becoming frustrated watching his head slip under the water, his methods proving to be ineffective. He wasn't getting better by anyone's measure. My patience was wearing thin. Dr. Treisman's words about mental illness being a biologically based disease gave me the strength and determination to parent James using what I knew was best for him.

James smiled a kind of grin, communicating to me he felt nothing but pity for me. If his smile could speak, it would have said, "You are not one of us. You do not feel the same energy I feel. Come, join me in this synchronicity that I feel with the earth, the people who lived here before us, the Penobscot Tribe. When I walk barefoot, I am connected to all of those who came before me and to all who will come after me." In his one persistent smile, I heard all of that. And I felt the trench deepen between us; the line between sane and psychotic came into perfect focus. There was cause for alarm and concern, but I had come to understand that unless I wanted to fall into the trench with him, I had done all I could to help him.

Leo, our large, white, eleven-year-old Italian Spinone, crazy with the smells of woodchucks, garden snakes, and other dogs who walked the trail before us that morning, took off down the wide path.

"So," I broke the silence James may have wanted to keep between us. "Looks like Isabella is gone. I see her car is not in the driveway." James was paying rent to live with three friends in a house on Thorne Street in Portland, but he was spending increasing amounts of time with Isabella at her apartment in Connecticut. Isabella was ten years older than James, and like him, she considered herself a "seer" and "visionary" because she too had experienced episodes of delusional thinking. They both agreed the goal of modern psychiatry was to support the pharmaceutical industry and that it was not in the best interest of the patient to take the drugs that purported to alleviate symptoms of what the Western medical world referred to as "bipolar disorder." They did not believe in diagnostic labels.

James had brought Isabella to Thanksgiving dinner in Baltimore six months earlier, and from what Daniel and I observed, she was a kind and compassionate soul who worked as an administrative assistant for a shipping company and lived in Stamford, Connecticut, in a tiny apartment on the second floor of a low brick building. She had brought homemade banana bread for me, a knit cap for Daniel to wear in the winter, and caramels for Julia and Nathan. With her long dark hair that fell to her shoulders, and deep brown eyes that matched the softness of her hair, she repeatedly let us know how fortunate she felt to be James's girlfriend. Sweet as she appeared, she did not help my crusade to keep my son on medication.

"Yeah, she took off early this morning," James said.

I nodded, thinking to myself how I didn't blame her. If I could have taken off at that moment, I would have. I craved my alone time and my walks with the dog by myself. These conversations with James tested my patience like nothing else he had ever done.

"What happened?" I asked him. "Why did she leave?" As far as I knew, Isabella had planned to stay for the weekend.

"Well, I had this dream about a woman I met at my Resistance Recovery group."

James's pace was slower than mine, so I stopped walking to be side by side with him. His step was steady, but he frequently chewed his thumbnail and pushed his fingers against his thumbs. His eyes darted from one side of the trail to another.

"What is Resistance Recovery? I thought the point was to recover. I'm so confused."

"It's a group I joined online. It's just a bunch of people who get together and tell their stories about getting off psychotropic drugs. We Zoom every Wednesday night at 7:00. There are a lot of people in this group, Mom, like hundreds. Anyway, I met this woman in the group, and I had this weird dream about her, and I feel like there is some connection I have with her. I told Isabella about it and let her see my text messages between this girl and me because I don't believe in secrets."

Leo darted ahead of us in the woods, occasionally checking back. Light dappled through pine tree branches. Daniel and I had done our research on bipolar type II disorder, and sure enough, hypersexuality, continuous affairs, and sex with multiple partners were common symptoms of a manic episode of someone with this disorder. To hear James talk about his interest in this other woman and then attempt to explain his actions to his girlfriend simply confirmed to me that my son was in a manic episode, proof of kindling for the fire I believed was burning in his brain.

More than feeling scared for James, or sad at the situation, I felt anger and frustration. Without help in the form of Western medicine, I saw no end to his pattern of establishing what appeared to be a close, trusting relationship with a woman and then making some egregious, unforgivable error that exploded the bond.

I sympathized with these women. "So you let Isabella know about your dream?" I asked him.

"Yeah, I mean my dreams are out there, you know?"

No, James, I thought. *I don't know. Your dreams are in your head until you decide to share them with someone.*

I didn't say that to him, either.

"Don't you think it's weird," he continued, "I mean, like, how everything is going on, like Black Lives Matter, the pandemic, don't you think it's weird how the pond water is so low right now? Whoa! Did you see those birds land on that branch?"

Instinctively, I paused and looked up at the trees, searching for the birds, but I didn't spot them. If James had been almost anyone else at that moment, I may have agreed with him about the state of the world and how it seemed like we were all walking around with knots in our stomachs. I might have acknowledged that it did seem like, because of the pandemic, people were empathizing with others more than usual. But because this comment from James followed other thoughts from him that made no sense, I didn't bother to discuss any point he may have been making, philosophically speaking. I was finished blurring the boundary between sane and psychotic.

He stopped walking and stared up at the sky, looking at the birds I never spotted, so I spoke to the back of his head. "James, I have no idea what you are talking about right now. You are not making sense to me. I really think it would be good if you saw a doctor, like a psychiatrist. You don't have to go on medication. Maybe you could just talk to someone."

"No, Mom. I know you don't see things like I do. I'm not gonna do that. I'm not going to a psychiatrist. I am feeling the disconnect here. Like, I know what Dad is up to on that internet board." He started to walk again, the soles of his feet turning a shade of greenish brown from the dirt and pine needles. Then he turned around and looked at me with an insistence in his eyes that said to me, You are not in my club. You don't understand me.

"James, what are you talking about?" He seemed to be off on a new kind of paranoia, one I had not witnessed in him before.

I was consciously confronting him with his delusions, which, according to every article on how to talk to a loved one about their delusional thinking, I never should have done. But I held out hope I could reason with him. He was standing right in front of me. This was my son. But was it?

"It's an internet company, Mom. Dad is telling you it's a pharmaceutical company, but it's really an Internet company that is trying to take over the world. It's run by a white supremacist and that's why you and Dad call the guest house the bunk house. Did you ever think of that? Believe what you will." He shook his head and gave a little pitiful laugh.

"James, Dad has been on the board of that pharmaceutical company for about five years. He is a biotech analyst. Why would he be on the board of an internet company?"

Leo stopped at the wooden bridge ahead of us, which connected Norton Pond to Megunticook Lake. James and I gazed down. Large rocks poked up from the lake, and I could assess the water level by looking at the wavy water lines on the rocks. It hadn't rained in weeks, and the water was unusually low. Maybe James was right? I leaned over the green-painted railings and tried to make my thoughts match the slowly flowing water. But despite my attempts to calm my mind and send soothing messages to my brain, my heartbeat was too fast, and tears gathered in the corners of my eyes. I admitted to myself there would be no reasoning with James at this point. I was walking the dog with someone who looked like James but actually was not James.

This was the third time in three years James had come to Daniel and me with disjointed thoughts and symptoms of a bipolar type II diagnosis that had gone untreated for too long. He sought refuge in us, his parents, and our home on the lake. But he stalked me with tangled questions, disturbing accusations, and thoughts that didn't make sense once they were out of his head. He spouted theories on Jungian synchronicity and Buddhism and banged rhythms on his drum, but when pressed for details about any of these philosophies, he would smile a maniacal grin, eyes flashing, and tell me I just didn't understand.

Talking to James felt like listening to a young child who assumes everyone knows the people and places he is talking about. Then, he was offended when I didn't recognize and condone the world he immersed himself in. Doctors and friends had advised me repeatedly to make a boundary, to protect myself emotionally. I remembered Dr. Treisman's advice to me: "If James were still using drugs, would you continue to support his habit?" I knew that by supporting James financially and providing food, shelter, and emotional support to him when he was delusional, we were paving the way for his pattern to continue. I played Dr. Treisman's words over and over in my mind, reminding myself that we were enabling James's belief that he could function without medication.

On this walk in the woods of Lincolnville, something in me snapped, and it snapped cleanly, like a dead branch from a tree. I was that branch, and I had hit my breaking point. I didn't want James following me on this walk anymore. I didn't want him at my house in Maine. I heard Dr. Treisman telling me it was okay to tell James to heal himself. I felt the need to protect my space in those woods at the lake that had always provided peace for me. I wasn't going to let him create chaos in my safe place. I turned from the bridge and started to walk back home alone. Leo paused halfway across, wondering why we weren't continuing around the lake like we always did.

"Mom, please! Let's just talk about our family," James said as he trailed after me.

The only sounds were the birds high above us in the pine trees, the occasional frog grunting from piles of leaves and squirrels chattering in the woods. I walked ahead of James and decided to take advantage of the opportunity not to speak to him. With each step, I planned out the words I needed to say to him. When we arrived at the driveway, I turned around toward him and broke my silence. I was not crying because I was not sad. I was not shaking, nor was my heart racing, because I was not nervous. I was sure of myself for the first time in a long time, and my words came out clear and strong, not a little like shouting.

"James, I can't have you here acting like this, not making sense. It feels hurtful. You are making accusations that are not true. Dad and I want to help you, but I don't think providing you with love and light, as you said you needed, is helping you. I need you to go back to Portland. You are twenty-eight years old, and I know that you'll do as you choose. If you don't want to take Dad's and my advice, I don't know how to help you. I can't do anything else for you here. I need you to go."

He stopped and stared at me, his eyes glistening. His right hand, fingers spread, rotated back and forth in the air by his hip in a way that looked unnatural and agitated. I walked down the driveway toward the door, and he turned and followed too closely behind. Yes, I was afraid that he was not in control of himself and would get physical with me or grab something in the garage and break it. He was my son, but he was a man now, bald like his father, brown-eyed like me, strong, and entirely capable of taking me down on impulse if he decided to do that.

I ran to the door, opened it, and closed it behind me. I was hot, despite the cool, late-morning air that had settled on the pond. I sat down on the wooden bench in the entryway, slid my feet out of my damp tennis shoes, and closed my eyes just for a second.

I waited for James to bang on the door, but he had not followed me into the house.

"What's going on?" Daniel asked from his seat at the kitchen table, his laptop open to email. He was probably on his second cup of coffee and wondering why I was sitting immobilized in the entryway. I realized I was not freaking out in my body or mind because, finally, I decided. I set a boundary, and it felt remarkably healing.

I walked up the three steps to the kitchen and looked out the window over the sink. I could see James headed back inside the guest house across the road. From the window, I saw him carry his drum and drumsticks to his car and watched as the blue 4Runner that we bought him on his sixteenth birthday took some dives in the potholes and disappeared around the first curve of Marriner's Drive.

"Where's he going?" Daniel asked, now standing next to me, staring out the window.

"Back to Portland," I told him. "I kicked him out. No, I didn't kick him out. I made a boundary. I can't live with him like this. He's making me crazy. I can't help him. One crazy is enough." Even though there was nothing else to see out the window, I continued to stare through it.

"Good for you," Daniel said. He had witnessed countless other moments when I had failed to make a boundary and my inability and unwillingness to do so had only caused more heartache for me and for Daniel.

I was relieved James was gone. I did not have to look into his eyes anymore, which felt like an emergency. I needed him gone. Just for a while. I hadn't felt safe in my own safe place, my home on Norton Pond. The feeling was scary, like looking down a tunnel with no way out, trapped in my own home.

Quickly, feelings of guilt swept over me as I stood with Daniel at the kitchen sink, gazing out the window at the path where James was no longer standing. Daniel put his arm around me, sensing my uncertainty. I asked myself, What kind of mother asks her bipolar son to leave the house in the middle of an episode? What kind of mother does not stand by her child in the worst times and offer unconditional love?

This kind of mother, I told myself. This kind of mother, who finally gets it through her head that unconditional love looks a lot like what I had just done.

STOP MAKING SENSE

JUNE 2020

Unlike other times in my life when I said yes but meant no, and despite Dr. Treisman's words bouncing around my brain like a ball in a pinball machine, I agreed to allow James to return the following weekend to the house at the lake in Maine because, from phone calls with him that week, and from talking with his friends in Portland, we gathered that he was not in a good place. We feared for his safety and, truthfully, for the safety of others. It was late June of 2020, and James had taken a leave of absence from a new job as a recreational therapist at St. Mark's Hospital in Lewiston because he found the job "unfulfilling," and his current view of Western drugs was in what he called "direct conflict" with what St. Mark's was trying to achieve with their psychiatric patients.

That Saturday morning at the lake, James sat at the kitchen table, gripping his cell phone like someone was trying to grab it from him. His eyes danced around the room as if he were following a tiny laser light bouncing around the walls. I poured him a cup of coffee, but he wanted tea again.

Okay, tea it was. I sat down in a chair at the table next to him and Daniel, where I could see the lake. It looked smooth and calm in a way that I was not.

"How are you feeling this morning, James? Any better?" Daniel asked him.

It would have been reasonable to assume Daniel and I had a plan of attack that weekend, that after speaking with multiple therapists and James's friends, and after having witnessed the increasingly delusional thoughts James was having, we knew exactly what to do next and how to handle James's illness. But I would be lying if I remembered it that way.

When you have an adult child who suffers from mental illness and who refuses medication, cohesive plans are difficult to make. We felt like our best course of action was to provide emotional support. To let James know we were always there for him but, at the same time, help him to understand that unless he saw a psychiatrist and followed medical advice, we didn't know how else to help him.

"Maybe a little. I just can't sleep. I took a Benadryl last night to try to sleep. I don't think it worked." James wore the same clothes he had on last weekend: dark athletic shorts, an old soccer T-shirt from high school, and tennis shoes. It all looked to me like it needed to be washed.

"You can take a nap later; try to relax on the dock," I said, taking a long sip of hot coffee.

James placed his hands around his mug of tea and positioned his phone in front of him on the table.

"What's with the phone, James? How about putting it away so it doesn't distract you?" Daniel suggested.

"I can't," he told us this with urgency. "Remember how I went to that Native American ceremony at Elizabeth and Paul's? Well, I took this homeless guy with me to Orono. Yeah, like, I was just trying to help him. I thought it would help him to be there. So I let him in my car, and he asked to use my phone, so I let him make some calls. When we were at Paul and Elizabeth's place, he slept in my car, and I think he may have done something to my phone. He masturbated in my car. I had to take it to get cleaned. But now I think he took over my phone."

"What do you mean he took over your phone?" Daniel asked him, as if masturbating in the car wasn't the clincher in that event.

"I mean, he tapped it. People are listening in on my calls, Dad. If it rings, I have to tell my friends to hang up, that I can't talk because he tapped my phone." James's voice was gaining in volume and agitation.

I glanced at Daniel, who was staring directly at James's eyes. This was going downhill quickly. I dreaded what the rest of the day was going to bring. I saw an emergency room in our future.

James went on with his delusions. "Dad, you know these pictures you have on the walls? You know your photographs? Don't you see it?"

"See what, James? What are you talking about?" Daniel glanced over to me.

The whole conversation felt surreal. The expression in my eyes must have communicated my fear as Daniel stood up and placed his hands in the air, just above his shoulders. The universal symbol for "enough."

"I know, Dad," James said. "You aren't where I am. These pictures are some white supremacist plots. There are weird things in these pictures, Dad. They all add up to things, you know?" James began pacing the room now very close to the walls, pointing out the photographs that were speaking to him.

Again, I thought to myself, *It's James's face and body, I recognize those brown eyes, I know that walk. But this is not my son.*

Daniel placed his hands on the table like he was about to make a move, but there was no move to make. We knew James would not check himself into a psychiatric hospital, nor would he consent to take medication. It was like a bad dream where you're in a math class, and it's the right room and the right teacher, but the final exam is coming up, and now you realize you haven't attended any of the classes leading up to the exam. I didn't know how to do this. No one, least of all my parents, had prepared me for the moment my child would slip over the line into a world that didn't make sense to me. I knew well how to coach him in soccer, how to help him write English papers, even how to make him feel better when he was sick with strep throat. But this? What kind of mother is prepared for psychosis? I wasn't.

"I'm gonna go swim in the lake," James announced and opened the sliding glass door that led outside to the lake. He walked out to the dock, leaving me feeling like I had already drowned.

Daniel and I watched from the large window in the family room as James pulled his shirt over his head, tossed it on a deck chair, and dove off the dock. Does cold water have the ability to place one's thoughts back in order? James swam from the dock to the middle of the pond, where he stopped and looked back at the house.

"I honestly don't know what to do," Daniel admitted, staring out the window. "We are going to get to a point where we can't handle him. We may have to call the police, and then he'll be forced to get treatment. I'm just telling you. I know you don't want to hear that, but it could come to that."

I knew Daniel was correct; it could come to that. And I would be about as prepared as any mother for that scenario to play out in my lake house. In the meantime, I would continue to believe I had some control over his treatment and that love and light may not cure him, but it also would never land him on the street. I would keep a-goin' with this kid until I couldn't.

Was there another choice?

MORE MADNESS

JULY 4, 2020

When James was not as tall as his fishing rod, his thin fingers used to pick through the mossy dirt he kept in a Styrofoam container on the dock and pull out blood worms. He'd bait the silver hook with the end of the worm so the worm dangled there. "Does that look good? I mean if you were a fish?"

He seemed to understand back then that if he reeled in his line too quickly, the fish wouldn't bite. Each time he caught one, he brought the fish into the boat without losing it. Most of the time, he didn't mind holding the fish above the gills while I taught him how to remove the hook without damaging the fish. James's reward, more fun to him than catching the fish, was leaning over the side of the boat and gently releasing the fish back into the dark, cool water.

"Bye, fish," he would say. "Maybe I'll catch you again."

The morning of Fourth of July weekend, 2020, James and I stood on the dock. The sun warmed the gray wood under our feet.

"I don't think I'm going to fish anymore," he said, his face smooth and tan, a black cap covering his head. "I don't want to cause anything any pain. I know you guys are planning to fish today, so I just wanted to let you know. I don't want to fish anymore." He stared out at the lake, his eyes dull.

"I understand," I said. "Sometimes I feel bad when we hurt the fish and can't get the hook out cleanly. Do you want to just ride with us in the boat? You want to wakeboard? The water might make you feel better. Come on, let's get you in the water."

I have always been one to get my children moving in the morning. My motto is "a body in motion stays in motion, a body at rest stays at rest," because this is the feeling I have inherently had in my body since I was a small girl. On this morning, I felt it was particularly important to get James occupied, doing something other than wallowing in his delusional thoughts. Maybe if he got moving, the adrenaline and the other chemicals in his brain would mix and bring my son back to me. It was an encouraging thought, although certainly not backed by any research, therapist, or doctor I had ever consulted.

"I don't know, Mom. It's like the water looks low in the lake. Do you really think you should be boating?"

I am sure I looked at him with narrowed eyes and a half smile. "I don't think the water looks that low, James, and I don't think that boating is going to hurt anything. We take the boat to the middle of the lake to wakeboard and water-ski. The water isn't low in the middle of the lake."

Why did I continue to reason with a person who was not thinking clearly? It was so tempting to take the bait; this person before me looked exactly like James, but he was not responding like James. These conversations with him were deeply frustrating and also just sad. I responded to the frustration by getting angry. My cynicism kicked in, and once again, I pushed him to do the things he used to do, as if running through the motions might remind him of who he was. If he wanted to hang around here, thinking this kind of rest, love, light, water, and lake life was going to treat his symptoms, then I wanted to see him try to help himself. And like my father before me, trying meant being productive, moving, and doing something to advance yourself. I would learn my lesson soon enough—I could not help James; I could not push James to be anything he didn't want to be. Only James could help James. But that July Fourth morning, I decided that if he was going to stay with us at the house and continue to refuse medical treatment, then he was going to literally join the crowd and jump in the boat.

"Mom! Don't you see it's all connected? You spill oil into the lake, the fish are suffocating, and the water level decreases. You won't have water to drink in the house if you keep driving the boat around the lake."

I looked straight at James's pleading dark eyes. He was serious. He raised his eyebrows, waiting for a reply.

But he wasn't making sense to me. Yes, fishing was not so kind to the fish. But we had a well on the property that supplied water to the house, and it was not dependent on the water level in the lake. And then I realized I was justifying all of this to myself in my own head. How many times would I allow myself to question my own sanity before I questioned his?

James and Isabella, who had since forgiven him for his dreams about the woman from his Resistance Recovery group, had been looking into and encouraging Daniel and me to wrap our heads around a therapeutic community in Vermont called Compass Rose, which purported to help individuals live with mental illness without the use of medication. Daniel and I had been adamantly opposed to the idea, based on the philosophy as well as the price tag. The program required a "seeker" to remain at Compass Rose for a year at a cost of over $100,000.

We told James and Isabella we were out and that if this was something James wanted to pursue, he had money in his savings account. It was intended to be used for his first house, or a car, or graduate school, but it belonged to him, and he could spend it as he chose. From what we had read about this program, it wasn't our choice of therapies for James. But something had to give, and we were becoming increasingly frightened about our lack of control and our inability to convince James to get into treatment, any treatment.

My younger son, Nathan, and his friend Matthew were at the lake for the holiday weekend, and they walked down to the dock then and stood next to James and me.

"Come on, James," I said. "Come wakeboarding. Show Nathan and his friend how it's done."

Nathan tossed life jackets into the back of the boat, then stepped in and sat behind the steering wheel and started the engine. Nathan and Matthew were sophomores at Georgetown University, lacrosse teammates there, and best friends since middle school. They held in their bodies a sense of confidence and invincibility, and Matthew's ready smile was difficult to turn down. Together, they created a momentum that said to me, "Let's goooo!"

James climbed in.

Daniel and I had been honest with our other kids about James's substance use disorder and his bipolar diagnosis. We told them everything we learned in real time. Julia was now a social worker who chose to stay close to James and was never hesitant to check in on him or to suggest to us ways to try to get James into treatment. Nathan's relationship with James had been more inconsistent—out of sight, out of mind when James was going through a bipolar episode, like this day. Having been through his own bouts of clinical anxiety and depression, and having experienced the relief that Western medicine was able to bring him, Nathan had little patience for James's search for treatment in drumming circles and meditation retreats. But here we all were, literally floating in the same boat. I untied the ropes from the cleats on the dock and pushed us off.

The propeller churned the green lake water, turning it white behind the Boston Whaler. Nathan cruised us out to the middle of the lake and cut the engine. "Do it, James!" he said, nodding his head toward his older brother.

"Okay, I guess I can do that," James answered.

I watched him pull the life jacket around himself and zip it securely. He took his hat off his bald head and placed it in the dry box. Standing on the edge of the boat, he paused before jumping into the water. He still looked strong to me, his calf muscles taut and his shoulders wide and broad.

Before he could reconsider, Nathan pushed him from behind, and James landed with a crash into the water. "Thanks, bud!" James shouted to Nathan, who loomed over him, warm and dry in the boat, and I saw a flash of the old James. As if jumping into a lake could unscramble one's thoughts, somehow place them back in order. Nathan glided the wakeboard through the water toward James, who slid his feet into the boots and tightened the straps. He had done this so many times, and it gave me a moment of joy that his fingers still remembered how to attach a wakeboard to his feet. To other people, it must have been like knitting or typing.

Nathan inched the boat forward, and the towline tightened in James's hands behind the boat. He appeared ready in the water, the wakeboard at the perfect angle for him to rise up, arms outstretched in front of him, fingers clutching the rubber handle of the towline. "Hit it!" he shouted, head bobbing in the sunlight, eyes ready and anticipating the next thing. "I'm good!"

If only, I thought to myself. *If only it could happen that fast.* Like some kind of holy baptism, he would be dunked underwater, and his thoughts placed back in order. My mind set free. All my worry washed away. How can you be good? I remember thinking then. How can I help you be good?

In an instant, he was up. He slid across the wake, jumped, and landed on the glassy water outside the wake. Back and forth he rode, a 180-degree turn, his left foot now leading. He shook his head to clear the water from his eyes.

Cheers, whistles, and hoots from Nathan and Matthew in the boat: "Whooo-hooo!"

Suddenly, James let go of the rope. He sank slowly into the water, as one does on a wakeboard that stands still. He floated there for a second, then removed the board from his feet.

"Why'd you drop?" I shouted to his bobbing head in the water.

"Tired. Just done."

He waited for the boat to come up alongside him and leaned on the wakeboard, breathing heavily. There seemed to be some urgency to his need to get out of the water.

Nathan circled the boat back, and James climbed up the swim ladder. Then he stood on the deck, dripping water from his athletic shorts and life jacket.

"Great job!" I smiled up at him. "You still have the moves!"

I said these words as if nothing was wrong, as if fifteen minutes ago, he hadn't tried to warn me about the dangers of drinking water from our faucets when the lake water was low, as if he hadn't told us his cell phone was tapped by a homeless man who had masturbated in his car. I said these words as if it were in my power to will him to be better.

"Yeah, it was okay." James looked at me like I had just made him perform some strange circus trick, but he no longer wanted to be part of the circus. He unzipped his life jacket and handed it to Matthew, who was going to try wakeboarding for the first time.

Then James took a seat on the bench in the boat, a green towel draped over his shoulders, leaned over the edge of the boat, and threw up. Brown bile heaved up in him, floating on top of the water. He lifted his head from the side of the boat, wiped his mouth with the back of his hand.

"Whoa, James. Are you okay? What brought that on?" I snapped back into my world of worry.

"I don't know. I feel my mouth get all dry, and then I get nauseous when I do something I know is against what I believe." He looked calmer now, talking softly, but his hands shook and he shivered, the green towel now dropped and drenched at the bottom of the boat.

"You don't believe in wakeboarding?" I knew what I sounded like. I knew exactly what I was doing. I wanted to shut down his illness, push it deep into this murky lake and drown it. I didn't want to hear about the damage boats cause to the water in the lake, or the pain fishhooks cause to the fish. This wasn't my son.

This was a video he had recently viewed on YouTube about theories of abandonment or Jungian philosophy. James's brain was like wet paint; every alternative theory someone threw at him stuck.

"Let's take Matthew for a ride, and then we can take you back," I told him, not yet willing to give in to his desire to get off the boat.

"It's fine, Mrs. Sandler. I can wait if James wants to go back to the dock," Matthew offered.

"No," I insisted, more to test James than to get Matthew wakeboarding. "Go ahead. Let's get you up on the wakeboard. You'll get up right away!" I was struggling to fully understand that James was not in his right mind, that he was not making decisions to purposely trigger me. I was operating on the assumption that he had more self-awareness than he actually had at this point. In anyone else, his behavior would be mistaken for selfishness, his words considered odd. As his mother, I might have risen above and given him a break, handed him a get-out-of-jail-free card. What kind of mother forces her mentally ill son to stay on a boat after he has just vomited off the side? I guess an angry one, one who is still clinging to the last fragments of the denial blanket.

When we returned to the dock, James moved slowly off the boat. Then he walked up the dock, past the fishing poles leaning against the chairs, past the kayaks and the paddleboards, and up the stone steps that led to the grass. He didn't turn around to check if anyone needed help with the towels, the ropes, or the equipment. He didn't say he would be back in a minute to help us put the skis away, and the life jackets back in the plastic bin.

He never looked back.

MY MODERN LOVE STORY

By Sunday afternoon, James left to go back to Isabella's apartment in Connecticut, Nathan and Matthew drove back to Georgetown, and I collapsed on the leather sofa in our family room, where I picked up the remote and hoped to be carried off into the land of insipid drama. I clicked on Amazon, and the *Modern Love* series popped up on the screen. Perfect, I thought, as daylight grew dim and the sky clouded over. I was a fan of the *New York Times*'s column, Modern Love, about relationships, and I sank deeper into the sofa, clicked Play, and stared hopefully at the screen.

In episode three, "Take Me as I Am, Whoever I Am," a woman named Lexi (played by Anne Hathaway) lives with bipolar disorder and meets a charming and handsome man, Jeff (played by Gary Carr), in the produce section of the grocery store. At first, Lexi appears to have it all: she is beautiful, charismatic, and has a gorgeous Manhattan apartment. She flirts with Jeff next to the oranges and lands a date in ten minutes. But then we see her depression hit her like an unexpected and unwelcome guest. She loses her job as a lawyer and hides her illness from everyone in her life, including Jeff. The episode closes with a shot of her, gleefully pedaling her bike, a brown wicker basket attached to the handlebars, down a busy New York City street. She looks radiant as she tells us, "I've finally accepted that there is no cure for the chemical imbalance in my brain, any more than there is a cure for love. But there's a little yellow pill I'm very fond of, and a pale blue one, and some pretty pink capsules, and a handful of other colors that have turned my life around. Under their influence, I'm a different person yet again, neither Madame Bovary nor Hester Prynne but someone in between. I have moods, but they don't send me spiraling into an alternate persona."

The room was dim by the time the credits rolled. I picked up the remote and clicked off the television. The screen went black, but I didn't move. James was not riding his bike off into the soft glow of the evening, reflecting confidently and affectionately about the positive outcome of his medications for bipolar disorder.

To have a child with mental illness was to live my life trying to stand on a ball. Sometimes I found myself shockingly balanced, wobbly but standing tall on the ball. Other times, I was completely off balance, falling off the ball, trying to figure out how to climb back on and regain my balance. It was, in some ways, James's ball on which I had to balance. Whenever he fell off, Daniel and I were called to pick him up and somehow, carefully and without the help of medication, place him back on the ball.

I thought about Lexi's parents and wondered where they were in this story of her mental illness. I imagined hugging Lexi's mother in a warm, understanding embrace. She would whisper in my ear, "Don't worry, dear. It will all work out."

"No," I would tell her, my hands on her shoulders, staring into her eyes, "James won't take the little pills that Lexi takes."

"Oh," she would say, her voice dripping with sorrow, stepping aside and forcing my hands to fall off her shoulders. "Then you will have to write a different ending to your *Modern Love* story."

IN PRAISE OF MEDICATION

I am not a doctor or a psychologist. I am a mother of three, but mental illness has been my stepchild, visiting regularly. My sister suffered from suicidal depression, my husband was diagnosed with bipolar type II disorder when he was forty-two, and my youngest son battled clinical anxiety in the form of panic attacks and bouts of obsessive thinking. My middle child, Julia, suffered from intermittent episodes of anxiety and depression into young adulthood. My maternal grandfather hung himself with a rope in my grandparents' garage.

Because of my experiences talking my children through episodes of anxiety, panic, and depression, and because I have witnessed the effect of medication on a tortured mind, I believe in the science of pharmaceuticals to give people who suffer from mental illness a break from their tortured selves. Yes, the mental health system sometimes fails. Patients get overmedicated in psychiatric hospitals, and there are side effects to psychotropic drugs. Still, it will be difficult to convince me these medications aren't life-changing when properly prescribed.

So when James informed us he was attending Compass Rose, a program in Brookline, Vermont, that claimed it could order his thoughts without the use of pharmaceuticals, it wasn't the program itself I feared or its pledge of "deep healing and safe tapering," nor was it the stunning price tag. It was the amount of time James would need to be there, unmedicated.

Approximately 55 percent of individuals with bipolar disorder refuse to take medication. According to the Mental Illness Policy Organization, "Although there is no cure for bipolar disorder, it is a highly treatable disease. The treatment success rate for bipolar disorder is a remarkable 80%." Experts in the field of psychiatry label James's emphatic belief that nothing is "wrong" with him as anosognosia, a lack of awareness that one is ill. In seeking advice and information about Compass Rose, James and his girlfriend, Isabella, referred us to Henry Reed, a therapist who lived in California. He had no degree in psychiatry, psychology, or social work, but he had written a book, *Harm Reduction Guide to Coming off Psychiatric Drugs*, and had been treating James for a few weeks before James and Isabella suggested the idea of Compass Rose to Daniel and me. "It is crucial to understand," Henry Reed wrote to me in an email before James left, "that drugs are drugs; there is no established disease process or mechanism of disease treatment for psychiatric medications. The drugs affect anyone who takes them as tranquilizers." I felt certain that he was ignoring the last twenty-five years of research on medication and the brain.

For the past few years, because of my uncertainty and guilt rooted in the possibility that I had somehow caused this disease to erupt in James, and because of my determination and belief that I could fix what I had somehow potentially broken, I read anything and everything on the subject of bipolar disease in young adults. Some of the journals were beyond my understanding without a degree in medicine. However, I was drawn to the first-person accounts, like Kay Redfield Jamison's *Touched with Fire*, and the memoirs by parents such as *This Fragile Life* by Charlotte Pierce-Baker, plus countless articles describing new research on the brain and mental illness put out by the National Institutes of Health in Washington, DC. I also read Henry Reed's book, and one given to me by James called *Anatomy of an Epidemic*, by Robert Whitaker, along with Whitaker's blog, *Mad in America*, whose mission states that his organization "serves as a catalyst for rethinking psychiatric care in the United States (and abroad). We believe that the current drug-based paradigm of care has failed our society and that scientific research, as well as the lived experience of those who have been diagnosed with a psychiatric disorder, calls for profound change." Whitaker is an award-winning journalist; his book won an investigative journalism award from Investigative Reporters and Editors.

And yet, I lived my research every day. Every morning for over twenty years, I woke up to my hypothesis about the efficacy of drugs and studied my experimental subjects, whom I lived with, and every night, I went to bed pondering my conclusions. I have rarely been so sure of anything in my life after witnessing the relief that psychopharmaceuticals brought to the lives of my own husband and children. I was not opposed to meditation, extra sleep, drumming, yoga, and any and all curative balms for the mind. In fact, I encouraged anything that felt good. I just believed that these practices needed to be in addition to the medication and not instead of it.

No one wanted growth and deep healing in the woods of Vermont for James more than I did. But I had little faith that was going to happen without a qualified therapist and a pill in a golden plastic bottle. It was my experience that the line between delusional and rational was real; of this I felt sure. Philosophically, in the world of *One Flew Over the Cuckoo's Nest,* I understood the overlap, but when you speak to a person who is having delusions, the line becomes obvious. James's request that we embrace this program as a means to whatever end he envisioned became too much for me to accept. Maybe sometimes we have to get angry at our children before we can provide the structure that will support them. It was like he pushed me too hard. I fell off the ledge, but I found my parachute.

FIRE

TINY CUTS EVERYWHERE

SEPTEMBER 2019

Daniel and I tried to slow the pace and hunker down at the lake. We put away the paddleboards and pulled up the dock. We placed tarps over the kayaks and wrapped new sapling trees in burlap, protecting them from the cold that would blow. But despite these rituals, we remembered. The remembering was like a cut on the bottom of my foot that I couldn't help but squeeze, just to make sure it still hurt. That fall felt like we had tiny cuts everywhere having to do with James. The cuts required our attention before they opened up and oozed again.

James spent increasing amounts of time with Isabella at her apartment in Stamford, Connecticut. We tried to accept Isabella for who she was, but I felt like I was holding a short piece of rope and she had ignited the other end. I held on until I burned.

That September, Isabella emailed me several times a day. The emails were disturbing to me, and I didn't know whether to reply or remain silent.

Dear Daniel and Judy,

You guys are going to make me cry (in a good way). I thought for sure I'd either not receive a response or your response would make me feel rejected, like, "Isabella, you're flipping crazy, stay away from our son or we will get a restraining order against you!!!" Thank you for being so freaking awesome and not doing that to me. I'm way out on a limb here, unsupported and this limb could snap at any moment but somehow, it hasn't. James does not know how good he has it with parents like you, and I'm not talking about money since money does not guarantee a good life. I'm talking about heart. Now I see where he gets all that heart from, you guys!

James was having an altered state crisis this morning. I gently guided diffused his "bomb" with more context and a story (based on Joseph Campbell's Hero's Journey). He was able to call and email Henry Reed (before acupuncture and therapy) but he has not responded to James's call/email as far as I know. Perhaps Daniel, (since Henry was so responsive to him) can take over on that front if James needs support in that area. Since James doesn't make a lot of money, Daniel might be able to figure out how to manage or request a sliding scale (or whatever you guys decide) since Henry charges $150/session if he is available for another client (fingers crossed). Besides if you ever read or watched any of Henry Reed's stuff, a part of James is just like him, but a few degrees/decades younger. The pairing of James and Henry is a multi-purposed idea that has sort of fallen in our laps when looking for ways to reach Samantha. Who knows? He could be a role model of sorts, etc. for James too.

Daniel and I pored over these emails. Over morning coffee, we took the sentences apart, line by line. This could be true; this is not true. Why is she saying this? Together, they seemed to be two mentally ill people who fed off each other's resistance to medication. Daniel and I took long walks around the pond in the late morning. By the time we got back to the house, we had received more emails from Henry Reed, from Samantha Clark, the director of Compass Rose. One afternoon, I got a phone call from someone who was on the board of Compass Rose. He told me he had a message he was supposed to be in contact with me.

"How did you get my number?" I asked him, still confused by why I was talking to this person.

"I honestly don't know. Didn't you call me?" he asked.

I paced behind our house, barefoot in the grass. I had an idea of who had directed him to call me and who had given out my number, but I never mentioned Isabella's name to him. "Definitely not, but I guess as long as I have you on the phone, I should talk to you about Compass Rose and my son." I gave him an abbreviated version of James's journey and what I knew about how we got here. I told him that I believed James's diagnosis of bipolar type II was an accurate one and that we continued to have faith in pharmaceuticals to control his symptoms. I tried to make it clear that I was not opposed to alternative therapies; they should just be done in addition to medication and not in place of it.

He shared with me his background and how he became involved with Compass Rose. He was chair of the Department of Integral Psychology at Burlington College in Vermont. He was experienced in the field of substance abuse disorder, and he told me about how he founded Plymouth House, a twelve-step retreat in Plymouth, New Hampshire. He was not opposed to medication, he explained, when absolutely needed. But he was a student of the "contemplative tradition," and he was interested in "how best to utilize wellness practice in place of drugs to treat mental illness." I listened patiently to him and tried to wrap my head around the possibility that any "contemplative tradition" could bring James back to himself. I wanted to believe him, but we were clearly talking from opposite sides of the mental health fence.

When I hung up with him, I was temporarily convinced that while Compass Rose would not be my choice of treatment centers, it was at least an attempt on James's part to acknowledge something was not right, and a shot at working to make it better. I did not wish him failure there, and I thought if he bought into the program, it might even work. But I had grown cynical of phrases such as "power of choice" to find your "inner balance" from Compass Rose's website.

Still, if James didn't find his peace somewhere, I was going to have to dissociate myself from him in order to keep my own sanity together. And who knows if I would be strong enough to build that wall between us? My past with James would indicate that I tended to poke holes in the walls I was supposed to build. That way, I could see him just enough to make sure he was okay. And we all knew what okay looked like—inky, like a stain I was having trouble getting out.

HOW ARE THE KIDS?

AUGUST 2020

Before Daniel and I climbed out of the car parked in front of our friend's house in Baltimore, I asked him how he wanted to answer the question, because we both knew it was coming. He was searching for the bottle of wine, which was on the floor on the passenger seat, in front of my feet.

Neither of us opened the car doors. We weren't ready yet to go inside for dinner.

"I'm not going to lie," he told me. "We don't have to go into every detail of James's latest episode. Let's just say he is struggling. Yeah, James is struggling. He is twenty-nine years old and struggling to find himself." Daniel sat up behind the steering wheel, the wine now in his hand. But he did not reach for the door handle.

"In the woods at a farm in Brookline, Vermont," I added from the passenger seat, just to complete the picture.

"Sure, if you want to tell them that. They're not going to ask for more details. They'll probably ask to pour you another drink at that point." Daniel stared out the front windshield. Tiny drops of perspiration formed on top of his bald head. He checked himself in the rear-view mirror, adjusted his silver, wire-rimmed glasses, and ran his hand over his smooth head.

"True," I agreed.

We opened the car doors, walked down the bluestone path, up the wooden porch steps, and gave a knock on the door. Kevin and Eliza were friends of ours, but we had not known them for long. Nathan and their son, Dylan, played on the lacrosse team at Gilman together. Daniel and I followed Eliza and Kevin through the kitchen and out to the porch through a side screen door.

"What a great porch! I'd never leave this spot." I was sincere in my compliment because I loved the wide, wraparound porch, and I would have had coffee out there every morning. Two white wicker chairs faced each other, and blue, down-filled batik pillows invited me to collapse into the chairs. A glass-top wicker table sat between the chairs, and a jute rug pulled it all together. Lush, green, hanging ferns made the whole thing feel healthy somehow.

"What can I get you to drink?" Kevin asked me, rubbing his hands together like he had a plan. "White? Red? A cold beer?" Smooth, tall, and somehow always tan, Kevin had a head full of salt-and-pepper hair, neatly combed and parted to one side. He was a successful fund manager and the kind of guy who still used words like "lads" when referring to our sons, as in, "What are the lads up to this evening?"

"Can you do a vodka and tonic with a lime?" I asked with a hopeful smile.

Then I waited for the question. The light was soft and warm, spilling onto the porch as if maybe there was someone up there who cared and was trying to deliver a message to me.

"I can!" Kevin said. "I like that in a girl. A vodka and tonic with a twist of lime is what you shall have!"

Daniel poured himself a glass of wine from the cooler filled with beer, wine, and ice. I sank into one of the wicker chairs, and Eliza sat across from me. She looked like a Swedish model—white, blonde hair blunt cut at her chin, and sharp, angular features. There was nothing willowy about Eliza Williams.

Kevin and Daniel leaned against the porch railing. I told myself I was a good liar, but I knew it wasn't true. I wondered if Eliza had secrets too. *Here it comes*, I thought, and I didn't mean the vodka and tonic because I was already holding that cold, wet glass in my hand.

I took a sip and readied myself with a believable, acceptable response.

"So, how are the kids?" Kevin asked, emphasis on the word "kids." "Bring me up to date." He was looking right at me, anticipation dripping from his wet, blue eyes.

There, he said it.

Parents of children who suffer from substance use disorder, anxiety, depression, bipolar disorder, or mental illness in general have two choices when faced with this question: lie and deflect the question, or be blatantly honest.

If I decided to lie and avert this hardball coming at me fast, I could speak in vast generalities and say, relatively speaking, all three of my kids were well. They had food on their plates, and they lived safely with roofs over their heads. They had parents who supported and cared about them. They were loved. And all that was true. But that didn't answer Kevin's question. I knew what he meant. He wanted to know specifics. Where were they working? What city did they live in? He wanted to know what their plans were for the future, whether they had partners, who those partners were. These are subtle subcategories hiding in the corner of the closet of the larger question, "How are the kids?"

But I find lying about how my children are doing more exhausting than telling the truth. I want to give people the benefit of the doubt and assume the statistic I had memorized like a soothing balm was correct. Chances are Kevin and Eliza had a family member who suffered from mental illness, or they knew someone who did.

"Kids are good," I told Kevin, with a tilt of my head. "Nathan loves Gilman; he's so glad he made the switch. He seems to be in his happy place there. Julia is living with her boyfriend in Denver. She's in her second year of graduate school at the University of Denver School of Social Work. Not sure how long they will live there after she finishes school, though; she tells us it's expensive in Denver. And James," I paused here and glanced at Daniel, raised my eyebrows, and gave him a half smile. "James is living in Portland, Maine, and is figuring out what he wants to do and what he wants to be. He is our struggling one, but he'll figure it out. We have faith."

I told this to Kevin with too much confidence, but I didn't lie. I nodded my head in agreement with myself. Then I looked at Kevin and threw that ball as hard as I could back at him. "And you? How are your kids? What are they up to?"

I didn't wish hardship on his children, but I wanted his words to drown me in empathy, instantly understanding through some secretly agreed-upon code what I meant when I said, "He is our struggling one." I needed to hear him tell me that his daughter was having trouble adjusting at Columbia, or that Dylan suffered from bouts of anxiety while only appearing to be the smooth, talented lacrosse defenseman that he was. I didn't wish it upon any of them. I just wanted to feel like I wasn't the only one.

"Kids are great!" Kevin said. "Kids are great." He glanced at Eliza, who nodded in agreement and smiled, then looked at Daniel and said, "Another glass of wine?"

TO TELL THE TRUTH

The words, "My kids are fine, how about yours?" perpetuates the lonely feeling of having children with mental illness and substance use disorder. Lying shuts the door and closes all the windows.

Mental health experts assure me I'm allowed to avert the subject. I am permitted to draw boundaries. Psychologists tell me to remember I alone do not shoulder the responsibility of carrying the weight of all mothers of children with mental illness. I have become an expert at flattening the details of my son's life. I say things like, "He's doing well. I mean, these are tough times for kids, right? How about your kids? Everyone well?" But when I do this, I can no longer hear what the other person is saying to me. All I hear is my own voice lecturing me in my head: *You didn't give her the benefit of the doubt. She might have a child with addiction issues. You could have shared stories. You closed the door and made it more difficult for everyone to talk about mental illness. You lied, and now one more person won't discuss this honestly.* Over 450 million people suffer from mental illness or neurological disorders at some point in their life. That is one in four people in the world.

Lying about how my children are doing at any given time preserves the stigma attached to substance use disorder and mental health issues. Secrets make my family lonely, and silence feels disrespectful to the incredibly hard work my children have endured in becoming resilient, empathetic, and wise adults.

I am no longer going to be that person who lies.

SUPPORT GROUP

OCTOBER 2020

At the advice of my therapist, I signed up for a support group for parents of children diagnosed with bipolar disorder. Because of COVID, the group met online on Wednesday afternoons from 3:30 to 5:00. They used to meet at a recreation center in Rockland, Maine, but it didn't matter anymore where anyone lived because during COVID, we just Zoomed. From the brown leather sofa in my family room in Lincolnville, my laptop on a low table in front of me, I clicked on the link and waited for the administrator to let me in the meeting.

It was 3:45 by the time I was allowed "in the room." There were ten of us there that day, ten small squares with ten faces in ten different places. I felt dissonance where there should have been connection. A man and woman who appeared together in one square took roll. They called each person by their first name. When they said, "Judy?" I replied, "Yup, I'm here."

The couple in the same square called on people, and each person explained what was happening in their life with their child or partner. Most of the participants asked a specific question at the end of their time—for example, "I'm wondering how to get my son out of my basement and into a program." One woman, a Nigerian mother of two sons, talked about her older boy and how he suddenly began to talk to himself and laugh aloud hysterically. He got violent with her when she told him she wanted him to see a doctor. Her younger son, in elementary school, tried to pull the older brother off his mother, and the younger child then dialed 911. The mother's question for the group was where to put her son after he was released from the psychiatric ward of the hospital in which he was currently spending mandated time. She was afraid to have him return home; her younger son was in school online due to the pandemic.

Another man in another window, maybe sixty-five years old, sat in a swivel chair. With his foot, he pushed himself back and forth, side to side. His son was forty years old, unemployed, and living alone in a townhouse. But his son seemed to move from one place to another, and sometimes, the man said, he didn't know where his son was living. How could he keep his son in one place?

"It's not good for him to keep moving from place to place," he told the group.

I would have preferred to remain silent and just listen, as it was my first time joining this group. But I heard the couple in one window call my name, and I felt like sharing stories was the expectation, so I spoke. "My son, James, is twenty-nine years old. He was diagnosed five years ago with bipolar type II disorder. He was on lithium and doing pretty well. He had a job as a recreational therapist at a hospital in Lewiston, Maine. Then he got involved with a group of people—well, a woman actually—who deeply influenced his beliefs about taking pharmaceutical drugs, and he stopped taking his medicine. He lost his job, and he has been cycling through psychotic episodes ever since. He is living in Connecticut now with this woman who is very much opposed to taking medication to treat mental illness. My husband and I want James to get back on the medication and return to his life. But he won't do it. He thinks he is doing pretty well." I paused and exhaled, forgetting about the question I was supposed to ask the group to consider. "Oh, right. I guess my question is: Has anyone had this experience of having a child refuse to take medication, and if so, how did you convince them to get back on the drugs?"

"Thank you, Judy. We'll certainly get back to you," said the couple in one window.

I listened to a few more people tell stories about their children. My eyes scanned each of the people in the windows.

I had the sudden urge to click on the red Leave Meeting button in the bottom right corner of my screen. If I were in a room with these people, I would go to the bathroom right now. I sought escape because I was scared, terrified really, that James would become like the swivel-chair man's son, unemployed and alone in a townhouse. I was scared he would run through our money, like several of these parents had confessed, and we wouldn't be able to afford to help him anymore. Scared he would never be able to hold a job, scared he would never be James again.

I forced myself to stay in my window. The group got back to me, and several of the people described situations similar to mine. Their children had gone off meds and refused to get back on them. I learned from the couple in one window about their daughter in New York City. She went off her meds, and in their opinion, she became a danger to herself and others. They got the court to mandate she take medication, but they had to forcibly transfer her to a psychiatric hospital. Apparently, that is legal in New York.

"Where is your son?" they asked me.

"He's in Connecticut right now. But he has a place in Portland, Maine."

"Oh," the woman says, "well, we don't know about Connecticut or Maine, but you could find out." I nodded, unable to speak.

I prayed it would not come to that.

At the end of the meeting, just like at the end of AA meetings, this group read from a script that appeared on the screen. Everyone read a line from the ten NAMI Principles of Support. When it was my turn, I read, "We reject stigma in ourselves and others." I thought about those words and wondered if I could ever actually give myself that gift. The couple in one window wished everyone a healthy week, then said they would meet next Wednesday at the same time. And then they added like a little joke, ". . . and the same place!"

I knew I wouldn't be back.

I might have returned if we were physically together. I crave connection with other mothers who have lived through this, but I couldn't feel the love from where I sat, hundreds of miles away from these people. I need, as I did when I sat in AA meetings when James was at Nature Quest in wilderness therapy, to feel I am not alone. I want to sit in an overheated church basement with people who, after dinner, make the effort to leave the house just as darkness set in outside, get in the car, and drive to the church. I want to sit in a room with thirty people and feel that my problems are not so unusual.

On my leather sofa with my laptop, I was still alone. Tears blurred my vision, but no one offered me a hot coffee in a paper cup. I clicked Leave Meeting and pushed the top of my laptop shut.

I am not like them, I thought to myself. *James will not be like their children.*

For an alcoholic, this kind of thinking is called denial.

A BAD JOKE

In order to apply to Compass Rose, one must complete a lengthy and detailed application process. In addition to the "seeker" spending a three-night trial at the facility, both parents and the seeker—that would be James—need to write their stories of his life. To me, it was like a bad joke: A mother, father, and son walk into a bar. The bartender says, "Hey, tell me the story of this boy's life." Which one are you going to believe? The only facts that Daniel's story and my story and James's story have in common are the date of James's birthday and how much he weighed at birth.

WE ARE ALL A LITTLE BIT CRAZY

But there is something called mental illness. Really, it's not up for debate among those who research the difference between neurological disorders and psychological disorders. Recent studies conclude that "neurodiversity" refers to those with cognitive and learning disabilities, such as autism, dyslexia, and dyspraxia, whereas "mental health disorders" fall into the categories of PTSD, anxiety, depression, and schizophrenia. No one wants to be a gatekeeper here, and certainly, there is overlap and room for discussion. However, there is a line I have to believe exists between delusional, mentally unwell, and sane, mentally healthy. For example, what if an anorexic person decided that anorexia was more a way of life rather than an illness? What if that person wanted to consider their way of life neurodivergent rather than an illness? Given that fatality can be a direct consequence of starvation due to anorexia, it is difficult to justify framing anorexia as a socially neurodivergent diagnosis rather than a medical diagnosis.

I would argue there is a line between the sane and the delusional. I know that James never killed anyone in a drunk driving accident.

His beloved babysitter, Anya, spent a lot of time with James at our house, but she didn't raise him; she never lived with us. Daniel's photographs were not hiding a white supremacist plot, and the water level in the lake was unrelated to the well that supplied the water to the house. I have trouble with James's use of the word "abandonment" in thinking about any aspect of my relationship with him. When James's delusions push me to the edge of my own sanity, the line between sane and delusional can feel fluid and transformable to me, but it is important for me to remember that it's there.

I WANT YOU TO KNOW

When working with mentally unwell people, let's say as your profession, I can see how it would be easy to diagnose someone as mentally ill. This person is not making sense, you might say, or, that person's behavior seems erratic. You have never known these people to be otherwise; therefore, you trust what you see. But when the person who needs to be diagnosed is your child, the one you have known—no, not just known, the one that emerged from within you, the being you touched and hugged, kissed, lifted, dressed, pulled, pushed, and held close to you, it is nearly impossible to, without warning, stop believing that what he says is the truth. I found that I would try anything, twisting his words around in my head like Silly Putty, to get them to resonate. Did the oil from the boat affect the water level in the lake? Was there another way besides the medication to cure him of whatever it was he wanted to call what was happening to him?

I want you to know that I tried. He almost took me to the edge with him because my love for him had no boundaries. And although love without boundaries sounds romantic, it's dangerous for all involved. But it was at this point in the story, reader—perhaps this is the climax, the point at which the conflict comes to a head—that a kind of anger set in. My brain turned into a flashing neon sign in a store window, only my sign wasn't flashing "Open"; it was flashing "Enough."

FROM JAMES'S APPLICATION TO COMPASS ROSE

JULY 30, 2020

I was born on November 25th, 1991, at Sinai Hospital of Baltimore, Maryland on Coldspring Lane. My parents resided at 1017 Windsor Road, and I was born 7 lbs., 11 ½ ounces. I grew up on Windsor Road and my best friend Christopher lived across the street. I was raised by my Nanny, Anya and learned to play chess from an early age by Anya's husband. There were many health issues and complications that I have difficulty remembering such as being born C-section, having a hernia, and my pediatrician consistently recommending drinking a lot of cough syrup for any cold-related symptoms I experienced.

PUBLICATION

JANUARY 2021

The act of writing is an exercise in creating one's story. Until I started to write this book, I didn't understand how tainted and one-sided our memories can be. It is a well-known fact that two individuals witnessing the same event may recall that scene using different and often contradictory accounts. The vagaries of memory depend on one's own identity, experiences, age, attention, and biases. I am my own unreliable witness to the events I most want to convey through writing.

For two years of a master's degree program, in which I received my MFA in creative nonfiction writing, mentors helped me understand how to tell my point of view and cautioned me against wading into James's story. I can't write James's story; that is for him to tell. I can only write what it was like to be me.

At about this time, in the middle of my MFA program and when James was about to leave for Compass Rose, I had a piece accepted by an online journal. I tell you this now because the event, and what happened after the piece went live, forced me to reckon with the fact that James, although still my son and still physically appearing to be himself, was not the James I knew and may not be that person ever again. What kind of mother, you may ask, feels anger about this realization instead of empathy? What kind of mother uses this heat like a lantern, to begin to find new ways to be with her son? This kind of mother.

A chapter from this book, "Did You Find Everything You Were Looking For?" went live on the website of an online journal in January of 2021. Two days after it was posted, I received an email from the editors that read, "At your son's request, we have removed the article from our website." Apparently, James took issue with many of the details of the way I remembered the story. Despite attempts to contact the editors and make my case, the piece remained offline, but I know now that when that piece was removed, James held up a stop sign for me. I admitted anger, I was embarrassed, and I needed to stop carrying on in the same way I had been taught by my father to "keep a-goin'." When James requested the editors take down my writing, my truth, my words, and my story, he effectively communicated to me that he and I saw his journey through two completely different lenses. And for the first time in my life, I realized that was okay. I was going to dwell on the conflict, thrive on my own theories, and believe, against everything I had been taught to believe, that I could love my son through this illness and hold my own story sacred. It didn't have to be the same as his, it wasn't going to be the same as his, and it was okay if we didn't agree on the rising action, the climax, or even the resolution. From where I sat with my laptop, we were never going to agree on those things.

FROM JAMES'S APPLICATION TO COMPASS ROSE

JULY 30, 2020

Sports were my saving grace in a way that helped me manage my anxiety and work through my emotional states and I excelled mostly in soccer and lacrosse. I was on vacation in Utah around new year's and was arrested, luckily only given a citation, and was not booked in Park City for possession of marijuana as the police in the area were allegedly looking for people who had been setting off fireworks. It was at this point that I did not know what to do and said I would try to get an old job working at Donnas to pay off the lawyer fees that my parents were more than willing to pay to clear up my legal record and make a case which eventually ended in a deferred disposition This led me to surrender my will to my parents and an educational consultant to recommend and choose a treatment center to address my substance use. I was blessed and grateful looking in hindsight to be able to spend 11 weeks at Nature Quest beginning on January 9th, 2012, learning "primitive" survival skills, camping, doing therapy, cooking on a fire, and walking the desert between the southern Utah and Nevada border. There, I was introduced to the idea of "skin walkers," and obsidian was all around. Many impactful letters and experiences were had and I was given limited options and chose to go to Alliance House in Portland Maine for aftercare. There, I began making roots in Portland and living out my madness without drugs and alcohol.

THIS IS NOT ABOUT JAMES

A woman I have known since I was a child, one of my very best friends, called me after my essay was taken down from the online journal. She has two children, one of them James's age. They used to play together in the bathtub. My friend asked if she could be honest with me, and of course, true to our relationship, I told her I expected her always to be truthful with me.

"I love your writing, you know that," she said. "I will always support you and what you write. But I have to tell you, I didn't like this piece. It was snarky. You sound angry and like it's about you, and James is the one suffering. I just didn't like the tone. I know you love him, and I do too. I love you, and I had to tell you the truth."

Her words felt like a bruise on my brain. What kind of mother publishes an essay about her child who suffers from mental illness, knowing the piece comes across as cynical? What kind of mother uses her son's mental illness as "material" for an essay, or even a book? I heard her, and I understood what she meant: a sad thing had happened to my son, and somehow, I was using my writing to try to make sense of it, to create something helpful to me and maybe to others experiencing the same thing. It came across as unempathetic to her and selfish of me.

But let me be honest and clear: That essay, and later, this book, were never about James or his point of view. I cannot write his story; I do not presume to know how he felt at any point in this story. I look for ways to tell my own truth to you, the reader. One of those truths is that to love a child with mental illness is frustrating, and sometimes, I feel angry. Angry that James asked to have my piece removed from the online journal, angry that I can't cure his illness, angry that he is not the person he used to be, angry because I miss that boy.

I didn't choose to write this book. It chose me.

FROM JAMES'S APPLICATION TO COMPASS ROSE

JULY 30, 2020

During my third year working at Oceanside Psychiatric Center as a recreational therapist, I was hospitalized at St. Mark's Hospital in Lewiston for thinking I had killed someone in a drunk driving accident and thinking I was a sacred clown and not eating or sleeping well. This elevated state of consciousness was brought about by being prescribed Effexor by my primary care physician and doing pranayama practice daily. I began working outpatient with a doctor through Maine Behavioral Health who would manage my lithium level via bloodwork orders and worked with me to only take lithium. I attended a session at valley zendo in Massachusetts two years ago and it really opened me up and was a major breakthrough and somewhat traumatic to be sitting with arisings and passings for four days in silence and 16 periods of zazen daily. Practicing zazen and attending retreats at the Monastic Academy taught by Shenzhen Young and Dr. Doug Tataryn has been a major development in my spiritual practice and depth. I attended some Native Institute workshops about Cherokee bodywork, hypnosis, and storytelling.

I'M GLAD YOU ASKED

"Maybe he's just going a different way.
Give him time, he'll figure it out."

I could tell them about the call from the cop in the middle of the night, sending him to wilderness therapy in the woods of southern Utah, the months of aftercare at Alliance House, what it's like to sit with him at AA meetings. I could tell them what I felt when I received phone calls from his friends who were worried about him "not making sense," or the time he called me and said he had killed someone in high school. I could talk about how, when you have a child who is checked into a psychiatric hospital, that fact takes over your brain like a balloon that just keeps filling and filling until there is no more room for any other thoughts. I could tell the story about having to pack his things from his house into boxes and plastic containers and bring them back to our house because he had acted erratically (read: irresponsibly and dangerously) with a woman and he was being evicted from the house while he was in the hospital. I could explain how, if you saw him, you would swear it was the same kid, the gregarious, outspoken, athletic person you knew as James, but that if you spoke to him, you would realize that person was no longer there. And I could brush off what some people say to me and smear their words across my heart like a balm or a band-aid.

"Maybe," I could say to them. "Maybe he will figure it out. Hard to know."

MY STORY

When I read James's application to Compass Rose, I shivered. My shoulders reached up to my ears, and I shook my head hard.

Anya "raised" James? She was our nanny from the time James was about two years old, and her daughter babysat for us frequently before Anya came to the United States from the Soviet Union. But they never lived with us, I never left James for longer than a few hours with either of these women, and I was stunned to read the word "raised" to describe his relationship with them.

He was given "limited options after leaving Nature Quest"? I felt rage at James's entitled phrase here. Maybe he forgot the price tag of a week at wilderness therapy? Or that we even presented him with a choice of places to go for his aftercare, despite the fact that we were thousands of miles away from him and it involved hours and hours of communication with his counselors in the woods of Utah?

He "surrendered his will" to his "parents and an educational consultant"? He was an addict, living in my house with his little brother and sister. We gave him an ultimatum: Get help or get out. He chose to get help, and we paid for it.

At first, when I read these things in James's application to Compass Rose, I was stunned, and I wondered how he could have remembered it all like this. Then, I just felt. I allowed his words and his point of view to sting me like salt water on open wounds. Maybe he remembered it all like that, but maybe there really was something wrong with him right now, something not right in his brain, and I was the one who was thinking clearly.

Yes, I told myself, it's okay to be in conflict with James. That conflict made me feel uncomfortable. But I believed I was correct.

THE NIGHT BEFORE COMPASS ROSE: TEXTS

AUGUST 4, 2020

JUDY: Hey Bud, I just want you to know that I love you and I will miss you. I wish you nothing but peace while you are there.

JAMES: I love you and will miss you so, so, so much. Peace and healing and health and help! Going to miss you and Julia and Nathan and Dad.

JUDY: We will all be here for you when you are ready to come back. Get everything you can out of Compass Rose. Do everything and be fully present.

JAMES: Yes, will do. Good night Mom, and sweet dreams. I love you and Dad.

JUDY: Goodnight Bud. Sweet dreams and Godspeed tomorrow.

LETTING GO

AUGUST 2020

The night before James left for Compass Rose, I lay in bed and closed my eyes, but sleep felt far away. I realized I would not hear his voice, receive emails or texts, or stare into his deep brown eyes for at least three months. He would not be sending me pictures or leaving me voicemails. If all went as planned, we wouldn't be in contact with James.

I felt my stomach go hollow. I pulled the sheets over my head.

Another part of me, up in my head, felt relief. I could exhale instead of holding my breath, as I had been doing for the last few months. Under the covers, I took a long, slow breath in and then exhaled. James would not be calling to let me know he had messed up the power grid for the city of Portland, and there would be no emergency calls from his friends, asking us what we thought they should do with him but letting us know that he was safe for the moment.

I tried to wrap my brain around the idea of Compass Rose; he would be safe there and part of a community. There were "guides" at this program and a psychiatrist on call, "in case of an emergency." I felt the warmth of my breath under the sheet covering my face. This could be a good thing. I reasoned I was handing him off to someone else for help.

"Here," I was saying to Samantha Clark, the director of Compass Rose. "You try for a while."

DID YOU FIND EVERYTHING YOU WERE LOOKING FOR?

AUGUST 2020

I had made this trip to Reny's before with a list in hand of one of my children's needs for camp or school, written in pen on a piece of paper torn from a spiral notebook. But this time was different. I folded the paper in half, made a crease, and walked into the store. I yanked a cart away from the others; I needed a lot of stuff today. My son had forgotten most of the things he would need in the woods, considering he would be away at Compass Rose for at least three months and possibly a year. It was August in Maine, and the air-conditioning in the store felt like relief.

1. Rain Boots

I scanned my options on the shelf and spotted a pair of brown leather Blundstones, low all-purpose boots for $150.00. Then I saw a pair of rubber black boots, size 8, for $22.00. I placed them into the cart.

"Can I help you?" A young woman with long brown hair approached me in the shoe aisle. Her pin, straight on her yellow work apron, said her name was Stacy.

No, I don't think you can help me, Stacy.

"I'm good!" I told her.

"Well, if you need help finding anything, just let me know." She returned to shelving shoes.

2. Tick Key

What even is a tick key? I picked up a flat piece of cardboard with a metallic yellow key attached to it. I saw it also came in metallic purple. James was good at picking ticks off the family dog with his fingers. He was never a squeamish child, loved to squeeze gloopy finger paint between his fingers, dig holes with sticks in the mud. At seven years old, I remember him groping around in a Styrofoam cup of worms. He pulled one out by its end and dangled it in front of his huge, brown eyes like a prize. "Put it on the hook," I told him. Guiding the worm, he baited his fishhook, a look of concentration and pleasure on his face. Whoever had written this list didn't know my son. He didn't need a tick key to remove a tick from anything. I threw the yellow tick key, whatever it was, into the cart.

3. Work Gloves, Two Pairs (One for Summer, One for Winter)

I tried to imagine James still in the woods of Vermont four months later, all the way into winter. Chopping wood, lighting fires, cooking, doing whatever he needed to do to stop the mania in his head. What size were his hands, anyway? His tiny hands used to fit inside my own, push Hot Wheels cars along orange plastic tracks, build LEGO airports. Then, they packed weed tightly into rolling papers and rolled them into smooth, thin joints. I thought his hands must have been medium-sized now. I threw two pairs of work gloves into the cart, one lined with Thinsulate and one made of black pleather.

4. A Journal and Colored Pencils

The last time I had purchased these items for James, he was starting fifth grade at Friends School in Baltimore. He had weaved through aisles like these—except at Staples in Baltimore—and examined planners, tossing into the cart fat pink erasers, spiral notebooks with holographs of skateboards on the covers. I had purchased it all for him, believing these things were a shield. That he would be bright and athletic if I checked everything off the required list. He was twenty-eight years old now and I was still buying him colored pencils. What would he do with these at Compass Rose? He would not draw giraffes that were mistaken by me for chairs, or sketch Egyptian temples for his fourth-grade project on ancient Egypt. I no longer believed I could save him by fulfilling someone's list of what they thought he needed. I tossed the pencils and the journal into the cart to buy them anyway.

5. Two Sets of Twin-Size Sheets

He had left without bedding. What was he thinking? He believed someone was listening in on his cell phone conversations and that the photographs on our walls were talking to him, so how could he have remembered to pack two sets of twin sheets? I couldn't bring myself to buy microfiber because I didn't know what microfiber was, even though it promised to be "soft and wrinkle-free."

I went with a blue damask print and a depressed maroon color. Before I placed the sheets in the cart, I remembered we had twin sheets in the closet at home. They were white cotton, with tiny blue anchors all over them. Anchors were happier. I also had a blue cotton blanket I could throw in. I realized I was doing it again, enabling James, doing everything in my power to make him comfortable. But I drew the line at microfiber sheets.

6. Sunblock

Despite the secret we all know now, that the chemicals in sunblock are more dangerous than the sun's rays, I stood before a colorful assortment of sprays and bottles. I was born before it was determined that the ultraviolet rays from the sun damage the cells of our skin. I confess to never wearing a drop of sunblock growing up, or even in college, and I confess to rarely applying it anywhere on my children's bodies. Even today, I will only reluctantly smear a few drops of it on my face in the summer. Get tan, boy, soak it up. Take your shirt off and sweat. Feel your muscles move. Get hot. Here's your sunscreen, but you know what I think. Check out this list of ingredients on the back of this bottle of sunblock. I was winking at him right then, literally closing one eye at the end of the aisle in Reny's. I threw into the cart this $5.95 aerosol spray can of sunblock. Just in case.

7. A Bathrobe

They didn't have bathrobes at the store. I asked Stacy, and she said they didn't carry them in adult sizes. On my list it said, "A bathrobe for the sauna." Since James was lucky enough to be taking saunas for the next few months, he could wrap a towel around his waist. Or Daniel had an extra bathrobe he could borrow. It had a Ralph Lauren symbol on it, and James wouldn't like that. What the fuck did I care what he preferred in a bathrobe? I had to stop caring so much. That may have been how we had gotten here to begin with—me caring too much. Now he was at Compass Rose, and I was pushing this cart around Reny's.

I rolled it to the checkout line.

"Did you find everything you were looking for?" Grant asked me, scanning each item I placed on the belt.

Everything I was looking for? I did not find the shelf holding the answer to whether three months or even a year at a place called Compass Rose in Vermont would bring my son back to himself. I did not find the rack where it was determined if an episode of bipolar disorder could be interrupted without pharmaceuticals. I could not find the aisle with the directions for how the saunas and the drawing and the work gloves at Compass Rose would quiet my son's brain and reignite his soul.

Grant, could you tell me where I can find these things?

SHENANIGANS

OCTOBER 1998

When James was in elementary school, there was a small, wonderfully crowded neighborhood toy store, Shenanigans, within walking distance of his school. At 3:30 in the afternoon, James darted out the door of the lower school's old stone building, his Buzz Lightyear backpack bouncing up and down behind him, some art or science project smashed in his balled-up hands. He crashed headfirst into my stomach, tossed his backpack at me, and asked, "Can I get a LEGO at Shenanigans? PLEEEEEZE?" I had no reason to say no, except for the mere fact that I should have said no to him more often. We had the time, and I could afford to buy him a LEGO every now and then. As it was, if I told him, "Not today," I was likely to get into a battle with a lot of crying and begging. Being conflict-averse, and fearing a scene at the carpool pickup line, I always said yes.

James scurried and babbled along next to me as we walked to the toy store, about how he sat next to David at lunch and that they played with beanbags in gym. He told me he didn't like his music teacher. Taking the back way to the neighborhood toy store, we passed the school's athletic fields, then the preprimary building on the left. We walked down a small hill, across another field, zigzagged through a parking lot, and then, recognizing where we were, James would take off into a sprint toward Shenanigans. Once inside, the owners, an older couple and their son, greeted James by name.

"Hi, James!" They would smile at him. "Got some new LEGOs in, want to see?" And the son of the owners would personally guide James toward the shelves where the boxes of LEGOs were stacked. James's wide eyes surveyed the tempting names: Luke Skywalker's X-Wing Fighter? Or, maybe LEGO City Police Chase at the Bank Building?

Sometimes James would circle the toy store at this point to make sure there was nothing else he wanted. There were cool things in this toy store; Shenanigans was no big-box toy store. The tiny space was crammed, barrels stacked to the top with magic tricks individually wrapped in plastic bags. Figurines of dragons, kings, queens, and soldiers lay in large baskets, waiting for little fingers to examine and choose them. Dollhouses and elaborate wooden castles, solidly built, perched on painted shelves. The sides of tempting and familiar games were visible from shelves just out of reach of children's hands—Operation, Clue, Sorry, Battleship, Monopoly, Guess Who, and Trouble.

Decisions, decisions.

Usually, at this point, now twenty minutes into the visit, James would reach for a LEGO set that even I knew was too expensive for a routine trip to the toy store, and I would tell him to try again for something smaller, which he did without too much grumbling.

While I paid for his after-school treat, be it LEGO or some new card game that we would later be trying to figure out how to play, James wandered around the store, handling everything he could reach, checking it all out for a future visit.

Immediate gratification always felt so easy and pleasing to me. As James sat in the back seat of the car, examining his new purchase, reading the sides of the box, every fiber of his being trying not to open it in the car, I drove home, imagining how the evening would smoothly unfold; James would do his homework on the family room table as requested. My husband, James, his little sister, Julia, and I would sit down to dinner, and for the rest of the day, until it was bedtime for James, he would be completely absorbed with his new toy.

In retrospect, I may have traded an afternoon of peace, or maybe years of them, for a lifetime of regret. Did my inability to consistently say no to James when he needed to hear it weave a fragile web of resilience in him? Did my fear of conflict build in James the scaffolding of his own fear of failure? What kind of mother can't see that children only get stronger when they are allowed to fall on their faces and fail? I would have had to be able to experience that myself to know it might be successful for my own children.

But my father saved me every time. And like a glass of wine, it always felt good going down. But oh, the hangover.

DANCING WITH YOU, HUNDREDS OF MILES AWAY

After I sent a large cardboard box containing the items James forgot to bring with him to Compass Rose, I received an email from Samantha Clark, thanking me for helping James out. Maybe this was the first time she had tried to save James, but I had been a card-carrying member of this party for a long time, so I was used to it. Maybe I was too used it. Maybe I needed to just stop.

I used to deliver his homework to his classroom when he left it on the kitchen table, and I spent hours searching for forgotten soccer uniform shirts and drove those shirts embarrassingly long distances on away-game days. I have been the class-snack mom and the help-with-the-homework mom, the mom who went in and talked to the teacher when James decided to be funny in class but the teacher thought otherwise. I have saved James a hundred times before. In his origin story, I am not sure which came first, his poor ability to plan and execute and follow through or my talent for taking over for him. Either way, here we were, the two of us, hundreds of miles away from each other, doing this dance again.

I'M GLAD YOU ASKED

"Do you feel like you weren't there for him? I mean, you didn't visit James in the hospital in Lewiston, and you sent him hundreds of miles away to wilderness therapy."

I could say that when he chose to go to wilderness therapy in Utah, I had two other children who deserved to live in peace. I could tell you he agreed to go to wilderness therapy instead of moving out of the house. I could say that outpatient treatment groups in Baltimore resulted in drug connections for him. I could explain that I was afraid of him at times because he had no respect for boundaries. I could say we had no choice. I want to say it was a privilege that we could afford to send him to a rehabilitation program that was out of state. I could say that, to this day, he is grateful for the chance to get sober in a community in the woods of southern Utah. I could say I felt the need to start making boundaries and that sending him to wilderness therapy may have been the first boundary I drew between James and me since he cried himself to sleep in his crib. That I had a job, a husband, two children, and a dog at home. I could say I believed he was in good hands at St. Mark's, that even if I flew to Maine to see him, I could only visit with him for two hours a day. I want to say that we spoke to him and his doctors daily and that his community in Portland was visiting him. I could say I am not just saying this, not just making excuses. I believe, even as I write this, that I made the correct decision.

"Do you feel like you weren't there for him?"

I almost drowned in my unconditional love for this kid.

BONFIRE

SEPTEMBER 2020

It was a clear, end-of-summer night in Maine, the perfect temperature to stand outside in a field, wrap my hand around a cool, brown bottle of beer, search out people I recognized at the bonfire, stop, chat, and move on. James had left for Compass Rose, and I hadn't written the no-contact rule, but I was enjoying it. I had not heard from him in two weeks.

I stared up at the sky, which was not yet black, still an inky blue. The fire burned in the shape of a tepee, sending orange sparks shooting into the night. The flames crackled and popped. My friend Lucas found me and stood next to me. We stared into the glowing center of the fire. He is a little older than I am, and we are good friends, the kind of friends where we both know to be quiet and just stare into a fire. Lucas knew what was on my mind. We had been talking on the phone, taking walks, sharing occasional dinners together. He broke our sacred silence.

"Carlos's brother is bipolar, you know." He speaks with a lilting Cuban accent that I want to listen to all day and night. His brown eyes glimmer when he smiles. Carlos, Lucas's partner of twenty-five years, is a doctor at the Pen-Bay Hospital nearby. "He still lives in Colombia. Carlos will be going at the end of this month to visit him."

I nodded, mesmerized by the flames, not wanting to come out of my trance. "How old is he?" I finally asked, wondering if there were any similarities between his brother and James.

"Oh, he's fifty-eight. He's been living by himself since Carlos's mother died last year. He used to be a tennis pro at a country club in Colombia. People loved him; they lined up to get lessons with him. But since he went off his medication, probably fifteen or twenty years ago, he has not had a job."

"James refuses to take medication, too," I say. "Why? Why do they refuse to take the meds?" I don't think Lucas knew how frustrated I was about this topic. I had told him a lot about James through the years, but not about how I worried every day that he would never take his meds again and never again function independently in the world.

"Carlos's brother goes around with taxi drivers now," Lucas continued, even though I was back to staring at the flames that licked the darkness. I was not sure I wanted to hear any more about Carlos's brother. "He drives around with them, and they take him to lunch way out in the countryside. They know where the best food is. We love it because when we come back to Colombia, his brother shows us the restaurants, and the food is delicious." Lucas kissed the tips of his fingers and opened them up like a flower. "But, his brother, he has no boundaries with people. Everyone is his best friend. That's how he meets the taxi drivers."

I smiled and let out a little laugh. This behavior, the issue with boundaries, I recognized in James. I told Lucas, "One time last December, James was visiting us, and we were shopping at that little gift store in Lincolnville. You know the one across from the general store? He struck up a conversation with the woman who owns it. I'm lucky she didn't show up at my house for dinner that night. What is Carlos's brother doing for money?"

"Carlos has set up a fund for his brother. He gives him enough to live on every month. Also, when his mother died, she left him some money. It's enough for him, you know?" Lucas told me this like Carlos's brother's illness was permanent. Like it's a done deal, and they have given up, which they have.

I was not smiling anymore. I took a deep breath and inhaled the smoke-blue air. "James is only twenty-eight," I said. "I feel like he will come around. Take the meds. He'll find out what he wants to do. I mean, at least, I hope he will."

Lucas nodded his head and stared into the fire, which I then realized I was standing too close to. It was making me hot.

COGNITIVE DISSONANCE

There's a name for what I have. I want to fall into the words like I would dive into a lake and submerge myself.

"Cognitive," as in, relating to the mental process of knowing or perceiving.

"Dis," as in, apart from, and "sonar," from the Latin, meaning "to make a noise."

"Dissonance": a harsh sound, discord, cacophony, sounds in a state of unrest and needing completion.

Cognitive dissonance is understanding the effects of Amazon on its workers and the environment but clicking "Order Now."

It's the sound of too many violins tuning up in a small room. The uncomfortable feeling of trying to hold two conflicting viewpoints in one's body.

It must have been cognitive dissonance I experienced when James first called me on the phone that weekday morning as I was driving to work and explained to me in detail an event that never occurred. He told me he remembered that he had killed someone in a drunk driving accident when he was in high school and that he knew I hired a lawyer to cover it up for him. He said he wanted to tell me that he was ready to make amends. I believed it was James talking to me, but it wasn't. This contradiction needed completing. It's dissonant.

Maybe cognitive dissonance explains the difference between how I remember James before that phone call—eager, funny, alert, quick, visceral, active—and how I have come to know him to be now—spiritual, slow, thoughtful, content, careful, introverted. It feels uncomfortable to try to hold both of these Jameses together in my mind.

Does cognitive dissonance explain the low buzzing sound in my head, like a swarm of bees high up in a tree, when James told me he didn't believe in Western medicine and that psychiatry was a field invented for the pharmaceutical industry? Could that be true? I think yes. Or no. It's cognitive dissonance.

Is it cognitive dissonance when you want to tell your son he can move in with you when he gets discharged from the psychiatric hospital, but all the social workers and doctors advise against that idea? How can it be wrong to take your own child back into the fold?

Because, cognitive dissonance, it is.

Cognitive dissonance is when I think of James as unmotivated instead of content, slow instead of relaxed, grabbing at straws instead of spiritual.

A therapist once advised me to grieve those things I can't find in James anymore. But I prefer to hold on to them and create within myself uncomfortable tension, a bungee cord stretched until it's going to pop back in my face, or cognitive dissonance.

At least there's a name for it.

A TICKING CLOCK

OCTOBER 2020

As the days that James spent at Compass Rose ticked off, I became increasingly convinced that I stood firmly in the company of people who believed in Western medicine to treat severe mental illness. There was a time when I would have stood up against anyone treating another person for anything against that person's will. But if you have not experienced trying to reason with someone who has anosognosia (lack of insight, an inability to understand and perceive that one is unwell), I beg you to withhold your opinion. Every day that James spent at Compass Rose, every day he did not receive medical treatment, felt to me like someone was turning a crank, ratcheting up my spine. I was just gaining momentum, collecting evidence, and waiting for Samantha Clark and her guides to make a wrong move with my son.

The three months of silence we were promised by Samantha Clark turned out to be very loud. Isabella repeatedly broke the no-contact rule, and then Samantha informed us James had found a way to slip a letter to Isabella by way of one of the guides. Samantha caved to what I know all too well to be James's relentless begging and gave him the letter from Isabella that was in the yellow envelope. James could be convincing and annoying in that way, but I felt Samantha and her staff should have known better than to give in to a seeker. The emails from Compass Rose arrived in our inboxes almost daily since the day James had left, and none reported good news. Daniel and I began to wonder where it would all lead. How would it end? My mind raced to the worst scenarios: we had been scammed, and he could lose his mind while he remained unmedicated. He could hurt someone; he might hurt himself.

Daniel, always the planner, brought up some very real possibilities: "Suppose he winds up being taken against his will to a psychiatric hospital, and he hasn't paid his health insurance in weeks because it is sitting at his house on Thorne Street in Portland? What if he leaves Compass Rose, goes back to Portland, gets his car, and kills someone on the road? Who knows when the last time his car insurance was paid?"

I began to wonder how a "therapeutic community" like this got licensed, or if you even needed a license to open up a group home and call yourself accredited. I reminded myself it was James's decision to go to Compass Rose, and I supposed I could have relinquished all responsibility, legally disowned him, and walked away.

But the emails were coming to us, and I couldn't sleep at night knowing James was in a delusional state and not receiving medical help.

IT HITS ME

I've told you: I don't like to get angry. It's not an emotion I was taught how to handle, so I try to avoid that one. Push it down inside my gut until it becomes an ulcer. But it is about this time in James's life, and it is at this time in my life, that I began to tingle with anger. I am not angry at James's condition. It's been too long, and we have come too far with him to continue to deny that he suffers from mental illness. No, I am not angry at his illness. I am angry that he will not help himself get better. I am angry that he has chosen to attend a program that I don't believe will help him in any way. I am angry that I have no control over his decisions. Nothing I do can keep the feeling away. I can't run enough miles, press it down into my gut hard enough, or talk to enough family, friends, or therapists. The dam is broken, and the anger is flowing through me.

AN ENTRY FROM MY JOURNAL

AUGUST 2020

Go to Compass Rose. Deep Healing Without Meds. Drum at their fires, cook in their kitchen, paint your soul with brushes at art therapy. Get your hands dirty in their biodynamic garden, chop wood, bend your body in a satisfying downward dog position, remember to breathe in, and then exhale slowly. Read, question, sing, dance, scream. Write the check for this program that one percent of the population can afford. Write the check every month for at least three months, maybe a year. Emerge from the woods of Vermont. James, you will be ready to do what?

IF YOU HAD BEEN BORN IN THE SIXTEENTH CENTURY

In earlier times, European cultures interpreted people who heard voices and saw visions, who had bizarre beliefs and broke with reality, as desirable people, and they may have been unusually blessed by the church. Many religious leaders reported hearing voices. But if those voices were sacrilegious or blasphemous, it might have led to a judgment that the hearer was cursed rather than blessed. Science has displaced religion as the established authority. But there is nothing that distinguishes mental illness from mystical experiences in the *Diagnostic and Statistical Manual of Mental Disorders*. Is science itself discouraging the extension of the human experience?

I think Samantha Clark would say yes. And while I believe there is room for all at the table, and I know that science may have its limitations in its understanding of the brain, there are no labels in the woods of Vermont. James was just another person who thought his cell phone was tapped and his acupuncturist was a Chinese spy. When he emerged from Compass Rose, he would have to operate in the world around him. He needed a basic reason to be, whatever it was—motivation to get on his feet in the morning. He had to be able to support himself financially, manage his health care (which was no small feat), and pay his bills on time. Maybe James was born in the wrong century. Maybe he could have been a high priest or a shaman, and other people would have washed his feet and made offerings to him. As it is, at this moment, I see him as mentally ill, walking around in a world that sees him as mentally ill.

A LESSON

James taught me many lessons, and I have been resistant to learning them. The lessons have been uncomfortable to take in, and the discomfort has changed me. With suffering comes pain, with pain, change, in order to escape the pain. It's a natural process. I am now a student of my own pain, and James has become my teacher.

I'M GLAD YOU ASKED

"But how, how did you lose the guilt, create boundaries, reckon with your past?"

I could say that when James was at Compass Rose, I had to slice through that codependent mother-son thing. I had to let it bleed out before it killed me. I could say I suddenly felt powerless to help him, or maybe I was always powerless to help him, but now that he was at Compass Rose, I wanted there to be space between us. I could say that I gave up if he was going to try to help himself by stepping into saunas and talking around fires. I could say, This is how I finally chose to help my son, by granting myself peace.

I will never fully lose the guilt, and my past is part of who I am. But to be at peace with James, I just need to accept who he is and admit I am powerless to save him. I admit that.

EMBERS

A NOTE ON CONFIRMATION

AUGUST 2020

Who doesn't need assurance? Who hasn't smiled just a little when someone told them that they were right? The emails that were flying back and forth when James was at Compass Rose only served to justify for me that, at best, James would take an expensive vacation at Compass Rose. At worst, the longer he remained off medication, the more damage would be done to his brain. And while I felt powerless to do anything about it, the emails from Compass Rose kept arriving in my inbox.

I wasn't sure how this would end, but I had a strange certainty about the fact that James's stay at Compass Rose was going to end, and also that it was not going to end well. But in the meantime, I admit I felt wildly confident and surer than I have ever been in my life about the danger that this program posed to my son.

So, with my husband, I replied to the emails.

THERE GOES THE OTHER SHOE

SEPTEMBER 2020

I didn't know what it would look like or sound like, but because I believe in science and the fine art of balancing medicine to control symptoms of mental illness, I sensed it wouldn't be long before I got an urgent phone call from Compass Rose. At the time, I was reading memoirs, journals, and scientific articles about psychosis, bipolar disorder, schizophrenia, treatments, and therapies. One disturbing fact popped up repeatedly in my research: The longer a person is allowed to be delusional, the more difficult it is to correct the delusions and get the person back to himself, whatever that might look like.

When I read this information, I felt out of control and desperate. Often an unrelenting optimist and can-do kind of person, confronted with this fact, anger set in. I was angry at myself for being so open-minded and believing against all probable odds that Compass Rose could help James. I was angry at James for wasting his money. I was angry at an entire alliance of people, beginning with Isabella and ending with Paul Jackson-Meade, for implanting cultlike ideas into James's brain.

For weeks, I was angry, and when I feel angry, instead of exploding, I am silent. It was just the way I was taught to behave in my childhood home. Rage, kicking, screaming, shouting—it got me nowhere as a child. I have since learned that the energy that it takes to be silent in the midst of rage escapes in the form of movement in my body. So I move. During the weeks that James spent at Compass Rose, I ran for miles in the late afternoon down our narrow street.

I ran the four miles around Norton Pond, and I ran through the woods with the dog. I swam in the lake from one dock to another so I had a goal in front of me. I took the boat out by myself, and, once I had steered the boat out of the pond and through the narrows, where it's shallow and "no wake" is the rule, I pushed the throttle to full speed and felt the rage drain from my body, like steam evaporating from a pot of boiling water.

When I finally pulled back on the throttle at the other end of the lake, my eyes were wet, and I heaved in large sobs. I cut the engine, let the boat absorb the wake of my speed, and allowed myself to be cradled and rocked on the water. Alone in the boat, I didn't have to be strong for anyone. I let myself feel the pain of James's illness and the anger I had toward those I felt were working against James's best interests.

My father had taught me to be numb in the face of trauma, silent when I wanted to scream. But I screamed on this lake. I screamed. And when I returned home, I would not be numb anymore. I would be the one who took control, the one who would find a way. Out in the middle of the lake, the boat held me afloat, and I could rage.

The call came from Samantha, right around dinner time. Her voice was kind and calm, and she told us not to worry, but James had been aggressive with another seeker. In her view, James was bullying this man and making his life miserable at Compass Rose. This man was deciding whether he wanted to stay at Compass Rose if James was allowed to remain a seeker. Samantha also reported that James was sorry for his actions and expressed that he wanted to stay and continue to do the work expected of him.

The following week, we received another call from Samantha. This time, she said James had bullied a guest who was trying out Compass Rose for his three-day visit.

A few days later, Samantha called to tell us that while digging up raspberry bushes and moving them to another site, James had thrown rocks at another seeker.

Finally, in what would be his last chance, Samantha called to let us know James had hit a guide on the back repeatedly after the man had turned around to do the dinner dishes.

It was raining shoes.

DO SOMETHING

SEPTEMBER 2020

Daniel and I fell asleep every night talking about what to do, what our options were, and asking ourselves, How in the world did we get here? When the pale orange glint of the sun rose over the lake, we opened our eyes, placed our feet on the warm wood floor, brushed our teeth, pulled on sweatpants and a T-shirt, and poured hot coffee into large mugs. We said the same things over and over again: There's nothing we can do. It's out of our control. He's going to do what he's going to do.

It seemed to me a harsh trick of nature that the loons continued to glide effortlessly around the dock, that the lake still lapped at the rocks on the shore, and that the sun warmed the gray wood of the dock. All of that would have to wait for us because James was our emergency now. It felt like he had been hit by a car repeatedly, but not only were we being forced to stand outside the police tape with everyone else, we couldn't even find the scene of the accident.

I was feeling all the feels, ready to act on James's behalf. All my mother-bear hairs were standing on end. I found it nearly impossible to "keep a-goin'" in the face of what I believed to be both poor and dangerous medical care. This is the story of a mother who shed her denial and came home to peace. Peace at this point in time could only be found through action.

I was desperate for someone at Compass Rose to take James to a psychiatrist for medication, to check him into a psychiatric facility. Daniel and I decided to compose an email together to Samantha, pleading with her to do something.

But before we could hit Send, both of our inboxes lit up with the other shoe.

From: Colleen McMillan
To: Daniel, Judy Sandler
Subject: Compass Rose Request

Daniel and Judy,

Unfortunately, James repeatedly hit one of our guides tonight. He crossed our line of "Anger is OK but violence is unacceptable" policy and therefore we need you to pick him up tomorrow. Samantha will call you in the morning to fill you in with more details, but we wanted you to know immediately so you could make plans accordingly.

Colleen McMillan

A NOTE ON OUR MARRIAGE AND IF HAVING A CHILD WITH MENTAL ILLNESS DIVIDED US

This book is not about my husband, my marriage, or even my relationship with my husband of, then, twenty-eight years. You will not be privy to the years of counseling sessions that Daniel and I attended together, separately, with James, and without James. I will not describe the waiting rooms, the magazines on the tables, or the sighing that took place in the waiting rooms. I will not write about the raised voices behind those doors, the tears, the blame placed, and then the apologies made, accusations taken back.

As of the writing of this book, our marriage has survived, and maybe even thrived, despite, or because of, these experiences. Did they affect our marriage? Of course, how could they not? Raising a child with mental illness placed stress on the weakest spots of our relationship. We were forced to shine a flashlight on the parts of ourselves we wanted to bury. How many times would he press the bruise? How many times would I shove him into the forefront because I didn't do conflict and I needed him to do the hard parts? Maybe we stayed together because we had this unspoken deal because we were able to see, despite the flashlight attempting to blind us. I would bruise but not bleed if he kept standing in front of me and throwing the punches.

TELL HER

SEPTEMBER 2020

I stood behind Daniel and read the email over his shoulder from Colleen McMillan, someone I had never heard from before, and shouted profanities I would prefer not to write here. I ranted about how I was sure it was illegal for them to throw him out of the program, and by "tomorrow" no less. I screamed at my husband, demanding to know how we could be expected to "make plans accordingly" when we had just received the email the evening before she expected us to "pick him up." I threatened to sue Compass Rose, sue Colleen McMillan, and swore I would put Samantha Clark out of business.

Daniel sat at the end of the table, rubbing his hand over his head while I walked around the table, repeating the phrase, "What the actual fuck?"

"You have to tell her," I shouted at him as I circled the table. "You have to tell her how out of line she is. She took James on as a seeker. I guess he's still seeking; she should know that. It was her idea to not give him medication, so now she can live with the consequences. He's a danger to others now. There's a law about that Daniel, tell her!"

Daniel pressed his lips together, looked down at his screen, and started a new email.

"What do you want to say?" he asked me, his eyes following me around the table.

"I just told you! Tell her we will not be making plans accordingly to pick him up from Brookline, Vermont, tomorrow. Tell her to please go fuck herself."

He shook his head and rolled his eyes.

We composed this email together, but it read a lot kindlier with Daniel behind the keypad.

From: Daniel
To: Colleen McMillan
Subject: Urgent

Thank you, Colleen,

I have received this email . . .

After conversations with psychiatrists, psychologists, and legal counsel in Baltimore this past week, it is clear to me that Compass Rose has accepted James as a patient and is now responsible for his care. While I do not want to blame your treatment algorithms for James's unacceptable and never before experienced behavior, I need you all to help us find a path forward for James since he has been in your care for the past month, and you arguably have a better understanding of what has caused this behavior.

Given that he is currently experiencing mental illness and appears to be a clear danger to others (rock throwing, hitting a guide) and himself, I would be in favor of your pursuing an Emergency Petition for Evaluation under Vermont's Involuntary Commitment Policy. I believe that he now meets the two prerequisites for involuntary treatment under Vermont Statute Title 18, Section 1701.

I strongly feel that we must apply a holistic approach to James's care combining appropriate courses of drug therapy to stabilize the genetic and physiologic underpinning of his mental illness so that your behavioral approaches can take hold.

I find it totally unacceptable that after accepting James as a patient and accepting our substantial payments for his care, you would now tell us that we need to "pick him up tomorrow." In my view, you and Compass Rose have made a commitment—moral and otherwise—and you can't just abdicate your responsibility on such short notice.

I feel that your unwillingness to provide medical management for James that may help him reach an equilibrium so that your behavioral approaches can work is putting your relatively narrow views on what proper mental health care is ahead of the need of a patient who is in crisis.

Sincerely,

Daniel

DRAW THE LINE

Samantha told us in emails and phone calls that she could not "force James to take medication." But actually, she could. She could have told him he couldn't stay at Compass Rose unless he took medication to stabilize his unpredictable and, at this point, dangerous behavior. She seemed to have influence over James, and she could have used her powers of persuasion to let him know that unless his actions changed dramatically, he was coming to the end of his time at the program.

But Samantha refused. Underneath her gentle and calm voice, that lilt of a British accent, was the strong philosophical belief that mental illness can and should be managed without drugs and psychiatric hospitals. This woman who founded Compass Rose as a haven for people to taper off drugs was not going to run too far down a drug-lined path with us, the one we saw as the only potential road back home for James.

There was an odd conflict going on in my body. The more times Samantha and Colleen reported James's "over-the-top" behaviors, the more confident I became that Compass Rose, and all of its claims of "freedom of choice," "deep and lasting healing," and "kindling of the divine and creative Self" amounted to little more than the tiny ember on the tip of a blown-out matchstick.

I had never been surer in my life of how to help James get back to himself, and none of my plans for him included any more days of chopping wood, farm-based work, alternative therapies, and biodynamic gardening. While it's true that only James was in control of his treatment plan, at this point, I felt like no one was in control of his recovery.

I had a strange sense that this was all going to come to an end in the next few days. And although I never wished more madness upon James, I could feel it in my bones that this was not the place where he was going to find his peace.

THE YEARS THAT ANSWER

"There are years that question and years that answer," writes Zora Neale Hurston. This would be a year that answered for me.

We form opinions based on experiences, biases, beliefs, judgments, family, and friends. If I ask myself how I came to the belief that James needed to be on medication, I will roll back time, rewind the movie, and unstack the dominoes. Flip the pages in the book backward, look at the pictures of him being escorted out of Oceanside Psychiatric Hospital, where he had worked for four years, talking to me on the phone that morning about the person he thought he had killed in a drunk driving accident. Play this movie back and notice there was a "before" he was on medication, a "during" in the time he was on medication, and an "after" he stopped taking his medication. My opinion about the value of psychopharmaceuticals to help those who suffer from a myriad of mental illnesses is based on my experiences, research, and discussions with psychologists, psychiatrists, as well as experts on the other side of the fence—Samantha Clark, Henry Reed, Isabella, James—and from reading

Robert Whitaker and Mad in America, and listening to *Resistance Recovery*.

I cannot deny their experiences. We live through the trauma and somehow come out the other end changed. We think we have the answers, but it's complicated. I can only write my story: who I was before James, how the experience of raising him changed me as a mother and a person, and how I came to hold the opinions that I do now. My beliefs are still fragile, but that's okay. That just means I am still open to hearing other voices. Those voices can't erase the video of my memories, and they can't delete from my mind the pictures I snapped along the way. The pictures are the illustrations to my story, the years that answer.

JENGA

Remember the game Jenga? You build a tower with fifty-four blocks and then take turns removing one block at a time. If you pull out a block and the tower falls, you lose.

That's what Samantha Clark's final ultimatum to James felt like to me. Only from where I stood, Samantha pulled out the last block. The ultimatum contained phrases like, *"Because of my aggressive behavior, which the Compass Rose community has tried to work with me for weeks, in order to remain at Compass Rose, where I choose to be, I am making the following commitments, or I will have to leave this loving and supportive community."* And, *"I will go outside if I begin to feel overwhelmed to avoid shouting at or being aggressive toward individuals. I will then seek support from a guide and work toward a resolution."* And finally, the last block, *"If they will not pick me up, I agree to go without resistance to the Rutland Regional Hospital. If there is an interim period, either I will remain separated from the seekers at Compass Rose or, with no resistance, I will go to the Colonial Motel or some other place."*

Asking James, at this point in his illness, to read, comprehend, promise, and be held accountable for his behavior was like asking a person who is blind to just try a little harder to see. It felt to me like Samantha Clark was offering James a trail of breadcrumbs to a place she knew he couldn't reach. You wouldn't tell a person with epilepsy to control themselves.

James signed the ultimatum while I awaited the call that would tell me they were taking my son to Rutland Regional Hospital. In fact, I would have welcomed that news. Her ultimatum to James had me seeing stars I never thought I'd see. I was not afraid of her, her staff, or the worst thing she foresaw in her contract with James. In fact, I wanted to make one more boundary. I emailed Samantha that we would "collect" James if it came to that, but we would be taking him directly for psychiatric care, and she should let James know to expect that, should we be called upon to pick him up.

I felt a strange calm washing over me. It felt like we were at the end of a thousand-piece puzzle. All the edge pieces were complete, and we were finally piecing together the middle of the puzzle. It seemed almost inevitable now. I thought I could begin to see what this puzzle was going to look like.

THE COLONIAL MOTEL, PART I

OCTOBER 2020

Samantha dropped the puzzle. The pieces were scattered, and I could no longer envision the whole picture. Around 7:00 p.m. on the evening of September 22, Joan, an administrator at Compass Rose, with whom neither of us had ever spoken, called to inform us that James had been dropped off at the Colonial Motel in Brattleboro, Vermont. Samantha would not commit him to the hospital; she backed down from her own ultimatum. Joan told us, "James refused to go to the hospital in Rutland, and we could not force him to go, as he is an adult. We really have no way to make him check himself in."

It takes a lot for me to lose my temper. I have been accused by my husband and children of being too generous, giving people the benefit of the doubt, always. But at that moment, it felt like Joan had struck some deep maternal nerve inside me. Whereas an hour ago, I had been waiting but willing to give Samantha Clark and her staff a chance, I was not playing anymore. I suspect Joan sensed this in the angry and cynical tone of my voice. "Joan," I said over speakerphone because Daniel and I were leaning over the phone again like we were looking for something in a toilet bowl. "You really think this is a wise decision? Let's think about what just happened. You took someone who you know is unstable and feeling desperate, who is still legally under your care, by the way, and you placed him alone in a motel room in an unfamiliar town. Let me just ask you one more time: Are you sure you want to do that?"

Joan told us she believed James should be on medication, at least to stabilize what she perceived as his violent and aggressive mood swings. She said she agreed with us that James should be checked into Rutland Regional Hospital. But it was true, she maintained, that James refused treatment, and short of having him arrested, which she knew Samantha would never do, there was little they could do to get him to commit himself.

Daniel and I listened to Joan's voice over the phone, glancing at each other on occasion, heavy sighs passing between us. When Joan stopped talking, Daniel dropped his head into his hands. Out of the large window that faced the water, I watched the neighbor's teenage boys dive off their dock into the lake. Their tan, wiry boy bodies glistened in the evening sun. *James was like that once*, I thought to myself. *He really was.*

I snapped my attention back to reality and the phone in front of me. "Joan, I hear you," I said, my heart beating wildly. I was not numb, and I could not pretend all was well with the kids. "But I am telling you, and you can let Samantha Clark know this; if anything happens to my son in that motel room before we can get to him, I will hold her and the entire Compass Rose staff responsible."

ENTRY FROM MY JOURNAL

OCTOBER 19, 2020

Rain finally. The lake is so low, the rocks expose themselves like dinosaurs emerging from the water. People who live around the lake tell me they didn't even know some of those rocks were there. Banks of mud appear on the sides of the lake, like beaches no one wants to see or wade in. But the sky opened up last night and steady rain banged against the roof and pelleted the windows. Last night I told Daniel, "I've done all I can do for him. If he kills himself in that motel room, I have to be at peace that I did all that I could do."

Daniel said, "We can't control him. He needs to make his own choices. If he decides to stay with Isabella, we won't leave him homeless, but we are finished trying to advise him."

We argued.

"I'm done," Daniel said finally at 5:00 in the morning from his side of the bed. He was lying face up, his eyes closed, arms crossed over his bare chest.

"You can't be done. It's too much for me to carry by myself," I told him.

I lay next to him, but we did not touch. I leaned against the white pillows and stared out at the fog lifting from the lake. I thought about what the water must feel like; secure and quiet, the opposite of Daniel's and my conversation.

Daniel said, "I have twenty-five years, maybe if I'm lucky, to live my life. I am not going to let him ruin every single day."

"It's not that black and white," I insisted. "You can't be all in or all out."

I did not raise my voice; it was too early in the morning for shouting.

"I can't be in the middle, remember? That's not me."

"You're going to have to be in the middle," I said.

"I'm trying." His eyes were still closed, but tears formed from underneath his thin eyelashes and dripped down his cheeks, making damp spots on his pillow.

Maybe he would fall back to sleep. It was still so early in the morning.

I could not even imagine what the rest of the day would bring.

WALGREENS

OCTOBER 2020

The name "James" moved across Daniel's iPhone screen. We were back at the kitchen table, leaning over the phone so we could both hear. James said he was at the Colonial Motel in Brattleboro, Vermont, and as desperately as Daniel and I wanted to drive there and rescue him, that simple, instinctual, gut-like desire went against all medical advice. Once we had James in our arms, what would we do with our possibly violent, unmedicated, delusional son?

We could not take care of him if he refused all treatment. Daniel and I agreed that if we picked James up from the Colonial Motel, we were driving him straight to a psychiatrist's office or checking him into a psychiatric unit in Portland, Maine. We had even contacted a friend of ours who was a psychiatrist on the unit to tell her we may be arriving that day with James. He had been in the motel room now for about twenty-four hours, and although we had spoken to him briefly, just to check he was alive, he had not agreed to our terms, and so I could not do what felt to be the most urgent and natural thing—go get him. It was a waiting game.

"Hey, bud, how's it going?" I thought this was a ridiculous question that Daniel asked, but what exactly was the correct thing to say to someone who had just been kicked out of a therapeutic living community and dropped off at a motel?

"I need to talk to you." James's voice was shaky, quiet.

"Are you ready to see a psychiatrist and follow medical advice, James?" I asked him. "Because if not, I'm sorry, but we don't know how else to begin to help you." I assumed he had hit his rock bottom and was finally calling us because he wanted help crawling out of the hole.

"Mom, it's not about that . . ."

"James, it's all about that," I interrupted him. "It's the only thing it's about. We can't help you if you aren't willing to try another path."

"No, Mom. Is Dad there? I need to talk to Dad."

"I'm here, James. We're both here. We're listening. What's wrong?" Daniel said.

"Dad, I think I got arrested in Walgreens."

Daniel and I looked at each other through narrowing eyes and furrowing brows. The dark wood table was still there, holding up the phone and scattered papers, and the bowls with milk from breakfast sat in front of us. The sun puddled pools of light on the water outside.

"You think you got arrested, or you did get arrested?" I could tell Daniel was trying to stay calm. The veins in his neck were beginning to pop out, and he scratched the side of his head in the way he does when he can't believe what he has just heard. His eyes darted around the room as if the answer to his question might be found on the sofa, the dog bed, or the rug.

"Well, I have a citation, and I'm supposed to be in court tomorrow. I mean, I look like shit. I look like I just came out of the woods of Vermont because, you know, I did just come out of the woods of Vermont. I mean, my hair is crazy long, and I have this big beard."

Daniel and I smiled at each other. It wasn't funny, but we had to laugh when we could. We shook our heads. This was what he was worried about. Let him be vain.

"It's okay, James. You can take care of all that. What happened at Walgreens?" Daniel asked.

"I mean, Dad, you know what's happening in this country, right? Like how the cops are arresting everyone? I mean, it's ridiculous."

My eyes drifted to the ceiling, and I thought to myself that the cops were not obsessively arresting white boys shopping at Walgreens in Brattleboro, Vermont. So no, I was having trouble following his thought process, but I did want to know how and why he got arrested. "Keep going, James. What happened?"

"I was just trying to ask for Benadryl capsules, and they kept showing me the stuff behind the counter, and I know you can buy it off the shelf. They were annoying me because I wanted the Benadryl capsules that are just on the shelf. And like, the next thing I know, the manager is asking me to leave, and I was like, no, I just want to buy the Benadryl. Mom, I haven't slept in so long. I was trying to get some Benadryl so I could get some sleep. It's really bad. So then the cops came, and they wrestled me to the ground, and like, yeah, they put me in handcuffs. It was really upsetting." James's voice trailed off. He sounded scared and shaken but not particularly sorry.

"Okay, James. You need to make sure you show up in court tomorrow. What time are you supposed to be there?" Daniel asked him. I knew he was trying to calm James down by focusing on the details.

"It says on this paper, ummmm, I think I have to be there at noon. Yeah, noon, I have to be at the courthouse."

"Can you get a haircut, shave, and some clean clothes? It's important, James, that you appear and that you try to sound sorry for your behavior. You really don't want this charge to follow you the rest of your life." I don't know why I said those words to James.

I think I was more afraid than he was of what tomorrow would bring. I grasped at familiar words, like "clean shaven," "sorry and regretful," and "the rest of your life," in hopes that these words would register something in James. But I was swatting at flies and missing them.

"Well, since I'm not allowed within four hundred feet of Walgreens, I can't get a razor. And I guess I can find some clean pants and a T-shirt. I have my stuff here."

"James, listen to me. Are you listening?" Daniel tried to stop the bleeding. "Find a barbershop. There must be one in Brattleboro. Clean up as best you can. Go into court tomorrow and tell them the truth. Tell them you were placed in a motel room by Compass Rose. Tell the judge you do not feel like yourself, you have not slept in several days. Tell them you became agitated, and you apologize for your behavior. Explain to the judge that you are seeking treatment. Can you remember that? Can you do that, James?" Daniel tried to place words into James's head, like a child sinking molds into Play-Doh. Maybe they would hold for now, but by tomorrow at noon, it could all be a sloppy mess.

"Yeah, Dad. I got it. Look, I gotta go. I'll call you back." James hung up and we heard the familiar sound of silence on his end.

Daniel and I looked at each other in disbelief. I raised both eyebrows. He had to go? Where would he possibly have to go? Maybe he had to make a few calls to "his people," who were advising him how to stay away from his parents who steered him straight into the halls of psychiatric hospitals.

WHY NOT SPEAK FRENCH?

OCTOBER 2020

Once again, Daniel and I were hunched over the kitchen table, a cell phone placed between us. Joan finally called; she was driving back to Compass Rose after court, and she had just dropped James back at the Colonial Motel. He had been there now for three nights and four days.

"How'd it go?" I asked. "Thanks again for going with him. We're really grateful you went with him to court." I sincerely appreciated that Joan took the time to accompany James. Whether she was directed by Samantha to go with him, or whether she chose to go out of sheer mercy, I will never know.

"You're very welcome. James already thanked me! I think he was glad to have someone with him. So, at first, because of COVID, the court made me stay outside the courtroom. Only the defendant and his public defender were allowed inside. But then, James spoke French to the court clerk, and he wouldn't answer in English, so they called me in."

Again, it was not a funny moment, but I had to laugh. Something about this was both hilarious and reassuring to me. I wanted her to say it again. Hearing Joan say he spoke French to the clerk was like a psychiatrist assuring me, amid all the uncertainty that swirled in my mind around mental illness, that yes, my son could be ruled "insane" by a court of law. James ignored all the advice he promised us he would follow, and in a courtroom in Brattleboro, Vermont, he answered in French to a court clerk.

"So," Joan continued, "after he began to speak French and refused to answer in English, they allowed me into the courtroom as his social worker. He was assigned a public defender. She's actually really great and helpful. She immediately realized this was a case of mental illness and asked the judge to withhold any decision until a court-ordered psychiatric evaluation could be completed. So that's where it stands. I took James back to the motel. I asked him if he needed anything, but he said he was okay, so I am on my way back to Compass Rose now."

Daniel and I looked at each other and shook our heads. Despite this astounding news, our mood was a little lighter; our path seemed suddenly illuminated.

"Look, Joan, we can't thank you enough. I know this took up an entire day, and we're so appreciative you stayed with James and also that you called to let us know how it turned out. We certainly wish you well. I hope we can talk again sometime." Daniel spoke sincerely to Joan, but I didn't think our paths would ever cross again.

If there are angels in this story, she is one of them.

With the knowledge that James spoke French when questioned by a clerk, I felt vindicated, like someone had pushed me back on a track and I was able to move forward again. The rails were greased;

the wheels were turning. I suddenly felt justified to help James in a way I had questioned before this incident. He crossed a line in my ever-expanding definition of mental illness, and with this new symptom, there was no question in my mind that he was unable to help himself. The path he had chosen to take to heal had led him to the edge of a cliff.

It was time to call James and get him out of the Colonial Motel. He wasn't going to live with us, but he surely could not stay there. This felt like a time of answers. For once, I knew what I had to do. So much of James's mental illness was floating around like dust on a windy day. Who knew how to catch it? Who knew if we should even try? But this decision to drive to Brattleboro, Vermont, and get him out of the motel room—this one seemed obvious and urgent to me.

PHONE CALL TO THE COLONIAL MOTEL

OCTOBER 2020

I imagined James sitting on the edge of a queen-sized bed, the small motel room dimly lit and beige. In my mind, he closed the curtains, the phone—the only thing standing between him and a way out of that place—pressed hard against his ear. I imagined his eyes: deep brown, a little wet.

"James," I said to him, hunched over the cell phone again. "Dad and I would like to come get you. You can't stay there anymore. We don't think you're safe. It's time to get you out of there."

"Okay," he agreed, all too easily. He sounded tired and ready to do whatever he had to do to leave the motel.

But this was James, I remembered, and I knew his fight was fierce.

"If we come and pick you up," Daniel continued my train of thought, "you need to agree to let us take you to either St. Mark's

Hospital for treatment, or to Portland to Spring Harbor. At Spring Harbor, we have already spoken to a psychiatrist who would be expecting you. You can't stay with us." I braced myself for his refusal; I inhaled, held my breath, and closed my eyes.

"Okay," he said. "I promise I'll go to St. Mark's and talk to someone about what I should do."

"No, James, that's not what we said," Daniel continued. "You need to promise us you will get in the car with us if we come and get you and go directly to St. Mark's and take the advice of the doctors. You need to promise you will cooperate and take the medicine they prescribe."

I inhaled again and stared out at the lake, which was quickly becoming one with the fading light. I was exhausted, and it was only early evening. A slow weariness crept through my body and seeped into my head. My eyes fixed on the water, and I let them close.

"Okay, I'll go with you," James mumbled into the phone.

"No, James. That's not enough," Daniel said. "Say it. Say you will get in the car with us. That you will be at the motel when we show up. That you will walk into St. Mark's with us and follow medical advice." Daniel looked up from the phone and glanced at me through his round glasses. He shook his head in frustration. I could tell he was about to snap.

"Yeah, okay. I hear you. I'll do it." Perhaps he wasn't as out of it as we thought. Maybe he knew exactly what he was and was not saying.

"No, James. Repeat what I just said. You are five hours away from us. We aren't driving to Brattleboro to have you disappear on us, or run, or not follow through on your promise to go to St. Mark's. You need to see a doctor. Then we can talk about what comes next." Daniel's voice was rising, and his jaw was clenched.

"Okay, okay. I will be here when you get here. I will go to St. Mark's with you in the morning. Can I please just sleep at the house for one night? I haven't slept in I don't even know how long. I just need to sleep, please, Dad?"

Daniel looked at me and raised his eyebrows. He silently shook his head no.

I begged him with my own brown eyes to allow James to stay with us for one night. We were so close to getting James to agree to get medical treatment. I talked to him without speaking. And because we have been married for thirty years, he understood my silence and read my eyes.

He relented.

"Okay, James. We are coming to get you tomorrow morning. You can spend one night at the house, and then we're taking you to St. Marks's. That's the deal."

"Yup. Okay. I love you. I'll see you tomorrow." And he hung up.

Daniel and I looked at each other as if in prayer, as if somehow our locked eyes could hold James to the promise we had both heard him make.

Who doesn't love a plan? It may not have been the one I wished for, the one where James graduated from college, found something he loved to do, fell in love, supported himself. Actually, it didn't even have to be any of that; I would have taken the plan where James just made sense. But for now, this was the map I held in my hand. It felt a lot better than the exhaustion of self-doubt and the panic of being lost.

YOU CAN CLOSE YOUR EYES

NOVEMBER 2020

My eyes were like a wall. If I kept them shut, I could forget that it takes five hours to drive from Maine to Brattleboro, forget we were staring down a ten-hour day in the car, forget I hadn't arranged for anyone to take care of the dog while we were gone all day and possibly overnight. My closed eyes protected me from my fear that James would not be in his motel room. While my eyes were still closed, I pretended James was good for his word.

Twenty-four hours later, to the minute, would prove that his promises were as valuable as leftover tickets to rides at yesterday's fair. The previous night, I hadn't even been sure we were going to do this, make the drive to Vermont. Daniel and I had still tossed around the idea of letting the rope go, of not getting sucked down the drain with James again. Of not going to get him at the motel. What would that look like? I think that was the last thing I heard Daniel say before I finally drifted off to sleep.

Apparently, we would never know. We were driving to Brattleboro, and we were leaving soon. Daniel shouted to me from the kitchen to our bedroom upstairs, where I remained under the satisfying weight of two blankets: "Can you grab an overnight bag and throw a few things in it for us? My toothbrush, some clean underwear, socks? We need to get going. It's five hours at least, you know? And who knows what we're going to find when we get there!"

I thought about how much I didn't want to move from my bed. But judging by the rate at which I heard him tossing papers around downstairs and arranging them in his leather case, gathering keys, and slipping on a black down jacket, I felt I should motivate. I dreaded this trip with every fiber in my body. I took a quick shower and wondered what would happen if we didn't drive to Vermont. Inertia kept me moving because I would have used any excuse to cancel this trip. I was in my father's numb place again, and it pissed me off because I knew better now than to go numb to protect myself, to allow my feelings to be tamped down like wet sand in a bucket. The problem was that if I felt anything right then, I was going to crawl back under those two blankets.

The anger I heard gurgling in my intestines would need to wait. The fear I sensed tingling on my skin would need to be melted by the coat I threw on my body before I left the house, and the sadness weighing on me about what James must have been feeling right then would all have to wait. It might stop me in my tracks later, but right then, I had to throw more clothes in the bag for fear this trip would take two days. I pulled another pair of pants off a hanger and tossed in a long-sleeve T-shirt. I dragged the suitcase down the steps and appeared before Daniel in the kitchen, hoping I looked ready to go.

"Ready?" Daniel asked, as if this could possibly be the start of some kind of fun adventure.

"Sure," I said, certain this was the only correct answer. "Wait!" I spotted the dog sleeping on the sofa in the family room. I could swear he knew when things weren't right around the house, and now, he lifted his head and looked up at me. "Hold on, I have to call Chris to let Leo out and feed him while we're gone."

"Do it from the road. Chris will be fine with it. Maybe we won't stay over. I just think we have to be ready, okay? I don't know what kind of shape James will be in."

James was the one suffering, but I felt angry and resentful. It wasn't just this trip that was making my blood run too quickly through my veins; that was just a smoke screen. Why was I really angry? I was angry at myself for being angry. I was frustrated that I had a child who couldn't save himself. I was sad that this is what it boiled down to. I knew better than to ask aloud, "Why me? Why my child?" but mental illness can sometimes feel to the caregiver like a selfish disease. That voice was noisy in my ears as we gathered the suitcase, jackets, and keys. But then, the numbness I had been raised on began to wear off, and real pain started to sink in.

My heart hurt that I was making this journey. I swallowed hard, my mouth formed a frown, and I felt a warm, sad hole in my stomach, like a huge tunnel that I was crawling through with weights on my back.

"Okay," I said, bending over to kiss Leo on his head.

I followed Daniel out the front door, climbed into the passenger seat of the car, and took an audible deep breath.

Maybe sensing my anxiety, Daniel attempted to pour some cold water on my sizzling brain. "Let's stop at Zoot, get some coffee and muffins, and then stop at the Market Basket and grab some of those good Sullivan Harbor sandwiches, with the nova and the toasted baguette." He put his hand on my knee. "Come on, we may as well enjoy the ride. Look out there! The leaves are going to be gorgeous!"

My body relaxed under the weight of his hand and the thought of hot coffee at Zoot. "I just can't believe we're doing this. I don't understand how we got to this point. How do you even get to Brattleboro, Vermont?"

I looked out the window as Daniel drove along Mountain Road and headed into town.

"I don't know yet." Daniel smiled at me. "We'll figure it out."

THE COLONIAL MOTEL, PART II

There was nothing colonial about the Colonial Motel. It was the opposite of what came to mind when I thought about a colonial building. Two low, dirty-white, faux-clapboard buildings arranged in an L shape in front of us as we drove down the driveway. A sign hung on a rusted metal post, directing us to bear right for rooms 200–225. We continued down the driveway until we dead-ended at a large parking lot. The building that housed James was across a wide expanse of grass with scattered patches of dirt. My nerves were spent. I had been in the car for five hours, but I felt the urgent need to get out of that driveway as quickly as we possibly could. There was something about the Colonial Motel that made me want to run in the other direction.

A woman and a small boy tossed a large plastic ball to each other on the grass. I wondered if they were living in one of these rooms or if they were taking in the sights of Brattleboro. A man dressed in dirty jeans and a dark T-shirt leaned against a building marked with a sign that read "LAUNDRY." He smoked a cigarette, exhaling steady streams of smoke out of his nose as he watched us lock up the car. I should have been excited to see James, and I should have been hungry since it was 2:00 and I hadn't eaten anything since early morning, but I was neither of those things. My heart was hammering in my chest so hard I wondered if this was what it felt like to have a heart attack. My legs moved without my brain telling them what to do because my brain was on autopilot.

What would we do if James wasn't behind door 205? Would we leave him here if he backed out of his promise to go to St. Mark's in the morning? Was it safe to bring him back to Lincolnville for the night, considering he had recently been expelled from a "healing community"? What would he look like? Would he be grateful and kind, or angry and resentful? The answers to my questions were just behind door number 205.

We stood outside the door, which was not wood, despite the deceptive wavy markings on the hollow, brown composite board. Daniel and I looked at each other and raised our eyebrows in one last affirmation that we were going to do this. He nodded his head. I knocked hard on the door but heard only silence. Each second that passed was terrifying.

Suddenly, the door opened and James was standing in front of us. Daylight cracked through the dark room. "Hey, bud," I said cautiously, standing beside Daniel still outside the door, resisting the urge to rush in, grab his stuff, and race away from this place.

"Hey, Mom," James said too calmly. He had a black, grizzly beard, and his usually smooth, bald head was covered in short stubble, like a crew cut that had grown out too long. A dirty T-shirt hung off him, and his jeans were secured around his hips with a red, orange, and cream macramé belt tied in a knot at the top button of his jeans.

"You ready? Can we help you get your things in the car?" I took a slow step toward the pile of suitcases, the duffel bags, blankets, jackets, and guitar, plus a large black and brown stuffed bear and a walking stick.

"No! I got it!" James told us. "Don't touch my stuff. I'll move it. Just hold on." He sounded disgusted, resentful, like we had come to steal his belongings.

I glanced up at Daniel, who was already holding a blue Southwest Airlines bag in one hand and a green backpack in his other hand. He didn't look like he was about to put the bags down, and he walked out the door with them, moving quickly into the light, across the grass and dirt, through the parking lot.

James appeared flustered and nervous, busy collecting bottles from the bathroom and jars of homeopathic medicines from the tiny, wooden bedside table. He washed these down his throat with a glass of water and threw other containers into a canvas bag, all the while shouting at us, "Just hold on! What is your problem? I'll get my stuff into the car!"

I was in fight-or-flight mode. My body wouldn't stop moving and packing because I sensed danger, and I felt like if we didn't get him out of there then, he might never come with us.

He was stalling for a reason, scampering around the room like a squirrel gathering nuts.

"Come on, James," I said in my best no-nonsense voice. "Dad and I have driven a long time. We just want to get you out of here and back to Lincolnville. I'm going to help you pack your things and take them to the car. Let's go."

I reached for the pale blue blanket that was tied up like a satchel around other blankets, sheets, and towels. I scooped up the bundle from the bottom and carried it, one arm over the top, to the car. The man leaning against the laundry building next door watched me, his head moving slightly with each of my steps. I passed Daniel on his walk back to the room to get more stuff. We made eye contact, shook our heads, and rolled our eyes. We rolled our eyes in solidarity, in misery, in some kind of silent agreement that we were hot, sad, and scared.

After three trips back and forth from his room to the car, we had James's belongings packed into the back of our 4Runner, and the three of us stood outside the car, staring at it. "Is that it?" Daniel asked James. "Do you need to check out? Have you paid already?"

"I guess," James mumbled in his best fuck-you tone.

"You guess *what*? You guess you have all your stuff, or you guess you have paid?" Daniel fired back.

"Both." James opened the door to the back seat, climbed in, and slammed the door shut.

Daniel and I looked at each other again, disgusted with our son. It was difficult to feel empathy, although it was probably what James needed at that moment more than anything. I have asked myself the question many times: What kind of mother feels resentful and angry at her son after coming to collect him from a motel room after he has been expelled from a therapeutic program and arrested in a Walgreens?

I was exhausted. My patience felt like a thin sheet of ice, and James was stamping all over it. I knew he was delusional and in need of medical attention. I see that now. And how empathy might have been better. But not only is there no visiting the past, I make no promises to myself about the future. Although the players will be different, the setting will be changed, and the script will not be the same, this scene will play out repeatedly. Sometimes I am empathetic, sometimes so frustrated I don't want to be with James. I have learned to forgive myself for all of those feelings.

Daniel settled into the driver's seat, and I sat in the front passenger seat. I glanced back at James. His eyes were already closed. He placed one hand on his heart, and the other rested in his lap. He maintained this position for the next five hours,

The memory of this trip is still stuck in my brain, much like an old photograph taped to the refrigerator.

TICKETS TO THE FAIR

NOVEMBER 2020

The next morning, James stood on the cold tile floor wearing only thin, black, cotton boxer shorts. His hairy, spindly legs poked out from pilled underwear. Gone were his long, defined calf muscles. Gone was his taut, tan stomach and the playful half smile from his lips, the smirk on his face, the glint in his eyes. He was too thin, and dark circles hovered beneath his eyes. “Come on,” he pleaded with me. “Just for a little while. I promise I’ll go to a psychiatrist and maybe talk about what drugs I could take.” As he spoke, he lifted his right leg and shook it out, repeatedly, while his right hand pulled at each of the fingers on his left hand.

“Come on, Mom, Dad, why are you doing this? Why are you in such a hurry? At least let me have some breakfast. Can I please have a cup of coffee? Let’s just talk about some options.” James still knew exactly how to rip at his mother’s heart until it lay bleeding on the floor for both of us to see.

But no, there would be no more talk. No compromises.

What I had to do was the antithesis of what felt natural for me to do. What kind of mother doesn't allow a child in need to return home? What kind of mother refuses to offer shelter and a cup of coffee to a son who has no place to go? This mother.

I was afraid to allow him to stay with us. We had to get him out of the house, and we had to do it right then. Daniel, who had been standing just inside the doorway listening, took a few steps toward James's pile near the bed. It was the same pile that had been on the floor of the Colonial Motel. We needed to get his stuff packed into the car again and get him out of there. James wanted to make a deal, but we weren't in the mood to bargain.

The uncertainty and the energy that it took to keep walking down the "tough love" path felt anything but warm and fuzzy. "James," Daniel spoke to him from across the room, "here's the deal. You either go with us to St. Mark's right now, or we take you to your car at Tommy's house. If you choose to go to your car, we don't know how to help you. Mom and I will be out of the picture. You will be completely on your own."

I still remember this feeling in my body. It's the same one I had when we gave James the ultimatum eight years earlier about choosing to go to wilderness therapy or getting out of our house. It felt to me now like when you know the right answer on the TV quiz show and you scream at the television but it's futile; the contestant can't hear you.

I tried to send James silent telepathic messages across the ping-pong table. *Come on, James. You know what to do here.*

He rocked sideways, picked up one foot, then another. "Dad, why can't I just stay here for a few days until I figure it out?"

One thing that has never changed in James is his stubbornness, his inability to surrender.

"Because that's not what you promised us yesterday when we picked you up." Daniel's voice was even, soft, and in control.

I wondered how long that lit fuse would last before it sparked. Daniel swept his hand from his forehead to the back of his head, then crossed his arms across his chest. I heard his body language loud and clear. Maybe James did too.

James said, "Fine. Take me to my car, I'm not going to a psych hospital. You have no idea what happens at those hospitals. I'm not getting locked inside some mental hospital, shot up with tranquilizers."

There was nothing more to say. We picked up his things from the floor, the same piles of towels, blankets wrapped around clothing, a walking stick, his homemade drum, his guitar, a suitcase of clothing, an unzipped backpack stuffed with T-shirts.

It was only 7:00 in the morning.

A CIRCLE GAME

In his early childhood, would it have made a difference if I had forced James to sit in his time-out chair, as his pediatrician at the time recommended? If I had said no to him on more occasions? If I had not been running beside him all the time, propping him up and saving him? Would he have developed more resilience and a better ability to understand how to help himself?

How about if we had not offered wilderness therapy to him but instead had kicked him out of the house? Forced him to "hit rock bottom," as addiction therapists recommended? All of these moments seem to me now like they might have been the big one, the one that would have made a difference in James's life. As if we had some control. I have come to believe we were just pressing buttons on a remote control that had no batteries. We kept trying to change the channel, but only James had the ability to recharge. From where I sit now, all these supposed pivotal moments feel more like a merry-go-round.

IS THIS THE BEGINNING, OR IS IT THE END?

NOVEMBER 2020

On the drive to Tommy's house in Augusta, where James had left his car while he was at Compass Rose, Daniel and I listened to James talk on his phone in the back seat. His conversations reminded me of when he was little and he sat in the back seat of our car with his friends and forgot I was driving, but I could hear every word. We knew that after he drove away from Tommy's driveway, he had nowhere to go. Isabella had told him that he could not stay with her, and we had made it clear that he would not be moving in with us.

On his phone in the back of the car, we heard him answering intake questions from a sober house in Portland. I gathered from his replies that, because he was not actively taking drugs or drinking, he did not qualify for their program. Then I heard James talking to his best friend, Sam. "Nah, I'm not doin' that." After that, I heard him speaking to friends of his who own a farm in

Buckfield, Maine, and from what I could gather from my seat up front, it sounded like they agreed to take him in for a specified number of days. I knew I wasn't supposed to care who took him in or where he wound up, but hearing James thank them gave me a shot of quick comfort, like stepping into a hot bath after a long, hard day. No longer numb, I felt fully present but gutted.

Tommy's house was in a neighborhood of neat clapboard houses perched on a small hill. Tommy was halfway down the cement steps before Daniel finished pulling up to the curb. He is a big guy, maybe forty years old, with brown shaggy hair and a warm smile. He gave James a bear hug and held on to him for a long minute. He shook Daniel's hand and gave me a hug too. I smiled at him and said, "Hey, Tommy, good to see you. Thanks for meeting us here." He helped us move James's things from our car to the back of James's car, which was parked at the top of his driveway. This felt like a moment to me, one of those big, pivotal moments. I didn't know when I would see this child again. If I stayed true to my word, the one that promised him I would be out of his life if he did not check himself into St. Mark's, then I had to let him go.

I stood on the black asphalt of Tommy's driveway, and tears burned in my eyes.

James reached out to hug me. "It's okay, Mom!" he said, as if, suddenly, he felt certain everything was going to work out for him. "It's like your writing, you know? It's like the beginning of my story. This is a beginning, okay?"

I stood in front of my son, nodding my head slowly. I peered out at him through my own brown, watery eyes that look so much like his. There was that thin, nebulous line again, the one that made me question who was sane here.

"It is, James," I said. "This could be a beginning. For both of us. Let it be a beginning, okay?" I hugged his thin body with everything I had left in me, and he hugged me back.

I watched him walk toward his car, climb in the driver's seat, start the engine. He smiled back at us and opened his window. Where was he going? I wasn't sure. But maybe, just maybe, I could trust that he knew.

ACKNOWLEDGMENTS

Portions of this work have appeared in previous publications. "I Confess," from a piece of the same name, was published in *Modern Love, Tiny Love Stories* (New York Times, 2022). "Scars" appeared in the Substance Issue of the *Perch* from the Yale Program for Recovery and Community Health (2024). And "Did You Find Everything You're Looking For?" was originally published in the *Awakenings Review* (vol. 10, no. 2, 2023).

This book has been years in the making, and it didn't look anything like this when I first started to write it. In fact, I didn't mean to write a book. Thank you to all my mentors at Stonecoast, at the University of Southern Maine, for teaching me how to write—not a book, just how to write: Suzanne Strempek Shea, John Florio (for the bricks and mortar), Ron Currie Jr. Thank you to the people who read the early drafts of this book and encouraged me to keep writing: #club57, Catherine Palmer, Jillian Hanson, Shannon Bowring, Nancy Hauswald, Julie Brown, Ricki Celentano, Mimi Edmunds. To Marilyn Moss Rockefeller, Elizabeth Garber, and Linda Buckmaster—what a privilege it is to write with you. Thank you to Andy Hanes, Jillien Lakatta, John Scott, Heidi Hutchison, Travis Henschen: I feel your love and support all the way to Maine. Beth Story, Emily Goldstein, Barbara Zadek, Fred and Cindy Beams—I am lucky to have you in my life. Thank you to Reneé Nicholson for seeing this book and making it happen, and huge thanks to Margy Avery, Kristen Bettcher, Kassi Roberts, Than Saffel, and everyone at West Virginia University Press. Special thanks to

Abby Freeland, Davis Shoulders, and Kendra Winchester for their energy, expertise, and patience with me.

There would be no book without Susan Conley. Thank you for believing in this book when I had stopped believing in it, for saving me, through the years, in ways you probably don't even know.

Thank you to my mom and dad, Marie, John, Joe, and Karen—I know you are there, and that's all that matters.

Thank you, Skip, for living the life we live with me and making it all possible. Thank you, Lucy and Noah, for your love and sense of humor.

Thank you, Alexander, for trusting me to tell my story.

NOTES

In her book, *Permission*, Elissa Altman writes . . .
Elissa Altman, *Permission: The New Memoirist and the Courage to Create* (Godine, 2025).

Epigraph
Ocean Vuong, *On Earth We're Briefly Gorgeous: A Novel* (Penguin Books, 2021).

I didn't recognize my own son . . .
"I Confess." In *Modern Love, Tiny Love Stories* (New York Times, 2022).

Never too old for that.
Judy Sandler, "The Caballeros Are Coming." In *Beautiful Things*, River Teeth's online magazine, September 7, 2026.

. . . and "Keep-a-Goin'," by Frank Stanton
Frank Stanton. "Keep a Goin'." In *One Hundred and One Famous Poems*, n.d.

. . . affects the part of the brain responsible
"Understanding Drug Use and Addiction Drug Facts," National Institutes of Health, 2025, https://nida.nih.gov/.

. . . genetic risk factors may account for half of the likelihood
Linda Armstrong, "Health Risks of Substance Abuse," American Addiction Centers, April 2, 2025, https://americanaddictioncenters.org/.

A cut that just won't scar over.
Judy Sandler, "Scars." In the *Perch* Substance Issue, Yale Program for Recovery and Community Health, 2024.

Did you realize you had an addict on your hands?
Peter Grinspoon, "If Cannabis Becomes a Problem: How to Manage Withdrawal," Harvard Health, May 26, 2020, http://www.health.harvard.edu/.

It's a mistake to think of one's life as plot . . .
Maggie Smith, *You Could Make This Place Beautiful: A Memoir* (One Signal Publishers/Atria, 2023).

In episode three, "Take Me as I Am, Whoever I Am,"
Terry Cheney, "Take Me as I Am, Whoever I Am." *New York Times*, January 13, 2008.

Approximately 55 percent of individuals with bipolar disorder refuse to take medication.
"Bipolar Disorder Manic Depressive Illness," Mental Illness Policy Organization, 2025, https://mentalillnesspolicy.org/.

"serves as a catalyst for rethinking psychiatric care . . ."
"Mission Statement," Mad In America, accessed October 9, 2025, https://www.madinamerica.com/.

She returns to shelving shoes . . .
Judy Sandler, "Did You Find Everything You're Looking For?" In the *Awakenings Review* 10, no. 2 (2023).

There are years that question and years that answer.
Zora Neale Hurston, *Their Eyes Were Watching God* (Spark Pub, 2014).

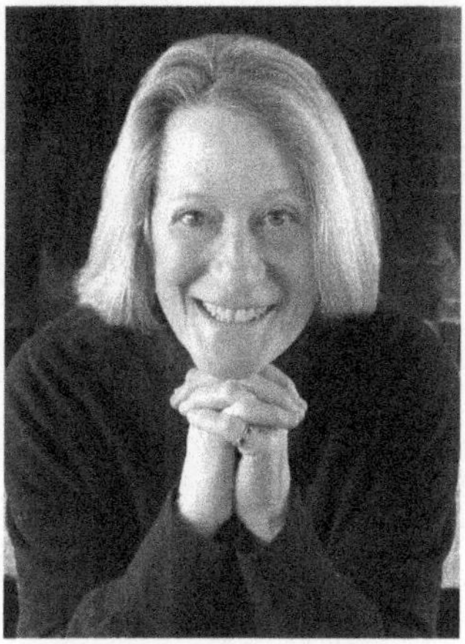

Photo by Harrah Lord

Judy Sandler is a writer and educator living in mid-coast Maine. She holds an MLA from Johns Hopkins University and an MFA from Stonecoast, at the University of Southern Maine. Her writing has appeared in *The New York Times's* "Tiny Love Stories," *The Atticus Review*, The Perch, Pangyrus, and the Treatment Advocacy Center blog. Sandler previously taught in Baltimore-area independent schools for over twenty-eight years. She is now the creative non-fiction editor for both *The Stonecoast Review* and *The Awakenings Review.* Sandler and her husband are the parents of three adult children, Alex, Lucy, and Noah.